D0906399

Basic Surgical Skills and Techniques

Basic Surgical Skills and Techniques

Editors

Sudhir Kumar Jain MS FRCS FACS FICS
Associate Professor
Department of Surgery
Maulana Azad Medical College and
Associated Lok Nayak Hospital
New Delhi, India

David L Stoker MD FRCS FRCSE
Consultant Surgeon
University College of London Hospitals and
North Middlesex University Hospital
London, UK

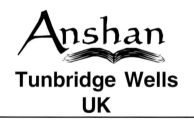

Tunbridge Wells
UK

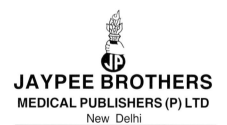

JAYPEE BROTHERS
MEDICAL PUBLISHERS (P) LTD
New Delhi

First published in the UK by

Anshan Ltd
in 2009
6 Newlands Road
Tunbridge Wells
Kent TN4 9AT, UK

Tel: +44 (0)1892 557767
Fax: +44 (0)1892 530358
E-mail: info@anshan.co.uk
www.anshan.co.uk

ISBN 13   978-1-848290-35-8

British Library Cataloguing in Publication Data
A catalogue record for this book is available from the British Library

Printed in India by Replika Press Pvt. Ltd.

Dedicated to

*Our wives and children for their
support in spite of their neglection by us during the
process of this work*

Our parents for their blessings

Our teacher for their wisdom

Our students who inspire us daily

our patients, from whom we continue to learn daily

Contributors

Amit Gupta
Consultant Surgeon
Vinayak Hospital, Noida
UP, India

Beryl Antoinette De Souza
Plastic Surgeon
Chelsea and Westminister Hospital
London, UK

David L Stoker
Consultant Surgeon
University College of London Hospitals and
North Middlesex University Hospital
London, UK

Gemma Conn
Specialist Registrar
North Middlesex Hospital
London, UK

Shiv Chopra
Consultant Surgeon
Indraprastha Apollo Hospitals
New Delhi, India

Sudhir Kumar Jain
Associate Professor
Department of Surgery
Maulana Azad Medical College and
Associated Lok Nayak Hospital
New Delhi
India

Vanessa Brown
Specialist Registrar
North Middlesex Hospital
London, UK

Preface

Apprentices in surgery need a basic set of practical skills in order to care for their patients well. Although many of these skills are same as those used by their 20th century predecessors, today's trainees need to keep abreast of rapidly changing and advancing technologies that were not available even ten years ago.

At the same time, basic surgical training for medical students and for junior doctors is being compressed into a shorter timeframe, as other medical specialties evolve and need to be taught in growing curricula. There is increasing emphasis on communication skills, and self directed learning in many undergraduate programs, and the student of surgery today has, therefore, to learn more in less available time. He or she will have less "hands on" experience in theater, ward or clinic and inevitably the practical aspects of surgery tend to suffer.

This small book aims to facilitate the more rapid learning required in a modern surgical program, with concise chapters on the main techniques that need to be mastered in the early years of training. It is intended to be read mainly by senior medical students, and housemen or interns, but may also be a useful revision for those about to take their first surgical postgraduate examinations.

It is the book written by working general surgeons to enhance the practical training of their own teams. It is also an international collaboration between London and New Delhi, and will be of use to students studying the art and science of surgery everywhere. It is not an exhaustive reference book, but more of a brief guide, to be used as a learning tool mainly in operating theaters and emergency rooms. It contains simple lists and diagrams with no superfluous text. There are clear explanations which should aid the student from scrubbing up to suturing up.

This book is designed to enhance practical training, and the student is encouraged to spend as much time as possible putting the basic skills described to good use in a clinical environment. Surgery remains largely an apprenticeship specialty, where only lots of practice will make perfect.

Sudhir Kumar Jain
David L Stoker

Acknowledgements

Our sincere thanks to Shri JP Vij, Chairman and Managing Director of M/s Jaypee Brothers Medical Publishers for his encouragement, support and inspiration. We are grateful to Mr. Tarum Duneja Director (Publishing) for helping us by valuable suggestions during the process of this work.

We express our gratitude to Mr Ravi, Medical Artist, Maulana Azad Medical College, New Delhi for making illustrative and informative diagrams.

We express our special thanks to the whole production team of Jaypee Brothers Medical Publishers for their hard work and professionalism, particularly Mr. Subrato for his help throughout the process of this publication.

Contents

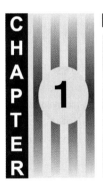

Scrubbing, Gowning and Gloving Techniques

SURGICAL HAND SCRUB

A surgical hand scrub is performed prior to donning a sterile gown and sterile gloves. Hand scrub does not render the skin sterile, but surgically clean, by reducing the number of organisms on the skin and hence reducing the risk to the patient if a glove is perforated during surgery.

Surgical scrub can be defined as a systematic washing and scrubbing of the hands and forearms with an effective antibacterial cleaning solution to render the skin of hands and arms as free from bacteria as possible.

The following two types of bacterial population are normally present on the skin.

Transient Organisms

These organisms are introduced on to the skin surface by soil, dust and by various other substances. Surgical scrub will remove most of these organisms.

Resident Organisms

These are primarily gram-negative and gram-positive bacteria with a natural habitat under the finger nails and in the deeper layers of skin, e.g. in hair follicles, sweat glands and in sebaceous glands.

Scrubbing removes bacteria from the skin surface and from just beneath the surface. After gloving, resident bacteria from the deeper layers are brought to the skin surface by perspiration and oil secretions, and the bacterial count on the skin again increases. Hand scrub therefore needs to be repeated between procedures.

Preparation before Scrubbing

Personal cleanliness is of paramount importance for members of the surgical team. This includes daily showers, frequent shampoos and attention to hands and finger nails. Staff with rashes, infective lesions or open wounds of the skin on hands, nails or arms should not scrub. Staff with colds, sore throats or systemic infections should not scrub.

Scrubbed personnel should have short nails, so that they are not visible over the tips of the fingers. Short nails are easy to clean and if kept smooth will not puncture gloves. Finger nails should be free from nail varnish, as chipped fingernail polish can harbor greater numbers of bacteria. Artificial nails should never be worn as fungal growth can occur when moisture becomes trapped between the artificial nail and natural nail.

Watches, bracelets and rings should be removed and kept in a safe place. Bacteria and dead skin cells accumulate beneath jewellery.

Every surgical team member should wear a clean, short sleeved cotton scrub suit before entering the semi-restricted/restricted areas of the surgical suite. Sleeves of the scrub shirt should be four inches above the elbow.

Street clothes or hospital uniforms are not allowed in these areas. A scrub shirt may be tucked in to the trousers to avoid contamination by the shirt tail flapping into the sterile field. Trouser legs should not touch the floor as this may transport bacteria from one place to another.

Personnel should wear shoes especially assigned for the surgical suite. Shoes should cover the toes completely. This is to prevent injury from sharp or heavy instruments falling from the operating table, and to prevent soiling of toes by the patient's blood or body fluids. Shoes should be cleaned at the end of the day. Street shoes are not allowed in restricted areas unless covered by sterile shoe covers. Shoe covers should be used on a single use basis and must be discarded on leaving the restricted area.

Personnel should wear a disposable surgical cap in such a manner so that hair is covered completely to avoid contamination of the sterile field by falling hair or dandruff (Fig. 1.1).

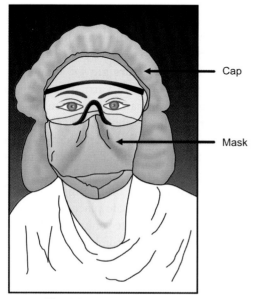

Fig. 1.1: Proper method of wearing cap and mask

A surgical mask should be worn by the surgeon, and assistant to cover the nose and mouth completely. This protects the patient from exhaled oropharyngeal bacteria (Fig. 1.1). It may not be necessary to wear a mask for all laparoscopic surgical procedures.

Environment and Equipment in Scrub Area

The scrub area should be large enough to allow the scrub personnel to gown and glove safely without hindrance.

A wall clock should be strategically placed to time the scrub, and there should be provision to control water temperature.

Sink height should be sufficient to minimize splashing, and taps should be elbow or knee operated.

Solutions Used

Hibiscrub—(Cholorhexidine 4%)
Betadine scrub—(Povidone iodine 7.5%)
Soap

These are in liquid form. The first two are preferred because:
1. They are non-irritating to most people.
2. They leave a minimum number of micro-organisms on the skin.
3. They have a prolonged antibacterial effect on the skin when used regularly. They leave a film on the skin which keeps the resident bacteria to a minimum and do not interfere with the skin's natural resistance to transient bacteria.
4. They lather easily in hot, cold or hard water.
5. The amount of detergent needed is small.

Scrubbing Method

Scrub should be performed before the first case in the morning and in between cases. Two methods of scrub technique are used, the time method and the brush stroke method. Rinsing time is not included in the total scrub time if the time method is used. In the brush-stroke method, a prescribed number of brush strokes are applied lengthwise for each surface of fingers hands and arms.

Unsterile objects should not be touched once the scrub process has begun. If this happens, accidentally, the entire scrub process should be repeated.

Scrub Up Technique

Scrubbing procedure must take a minimum of two minutes if scrub solutions are used and five minutes if soap is used.

Water temperature should be set at comfort level.

Wet hands and forearms (Fig. 1.2).

Dispense around 5 ml of antibacterial soap solution in to the palm. A nail brush should be used only on nails or in web spaces but not on rest of the skin (Fig. 1.3).

Scrubbing should start from fingers to one inch below the elbow, not from elbow to fingers (Fig. 1.4).

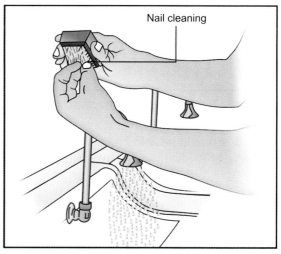

Fig. 1.3: Scrub finger nails with nail brush

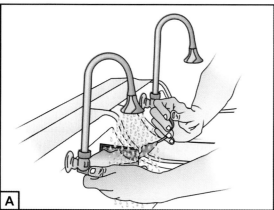

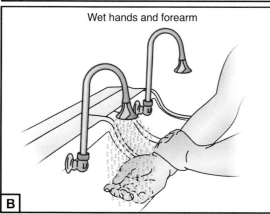

Figs 1.2A and B: Wet hands and forearms before starting scrub

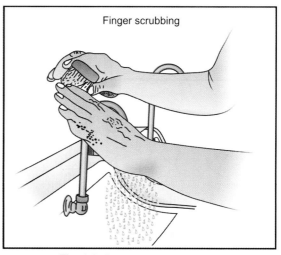

Fig. 1.4: Scrub all sides of fingers

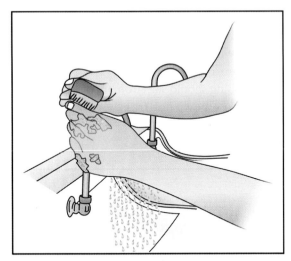

Fig. 1.5: Continuing scrub process on hands

Hands should be held higher than elbow, so that water flows downwards off the elbows (Fig. 1.5).

Water splashing on theater clothes should be avoided as wet clothes may cause contamination of the sterile gown. Hands and forearms should be washed and rinsed at least twice after scrubbing (Fig. 1.6).

Following the final rinse, the hands and forearms should be elevated away from the body allowing water to drop from the elbows. Hands and forearms should be dried using a folded disposable hand towel separately for each side. Drying should start from fingers towards elbows. The towels should be discarded immediately after drying the hands and forearm. Towel should remain folded to double thickness while drying (Figs 1.7 to 1.10).

Surgical Gown Technique

Gowns should be properly fitting, permitting freedom of movement. Each sleeve should be provided with a tight fitting cuff. Gowns should ideally be water repellent.

When donning a gown one should touch only the inside surface. If the outside of the gown is touched, it is deemed contaminated and should be discarded. Gowns are folded with the inside facing the scrubbed person to facilitate sterile gowning.

Scrubbed personnel should keep their hands and arms above their waist and away from the

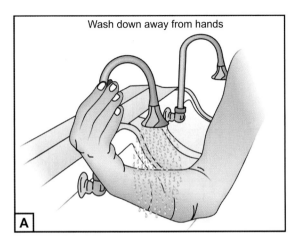

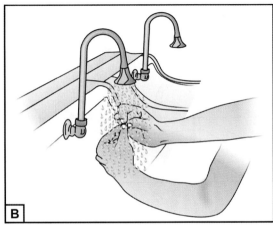

Figs 1.6A and B: Rinsing forearms and hands

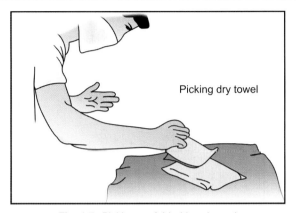

Fig. 1.7: Picking up folded hand towel

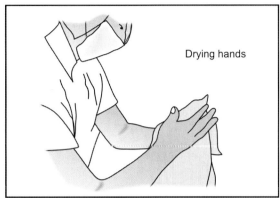

Fig. 1.8: Drying hands using rotating movements

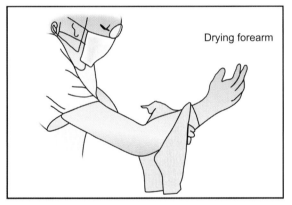

Fig. 1.9: Drying the forearms

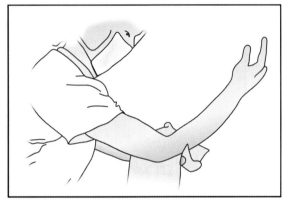

Fig. 1.10: Drying the elbows

body at an angle of 20 to 30° above the elbows. If scrubbed hands and arms fall below waist level they are considered contaminated.

After donning, the parts which are considered sterile are sleeves (except the axillary area) and the front from waist level to a few inches below the neck opening. Gowns must be made of material that minimizes the passage of micro-organisms and body fluids, and should also be tear and puncture resistant. They should be lint free to reduce particle dissemination into the wound or the environment.

Procedure for Gowning

Lift the inner side of the neck of the gown upwards and away from the table (Fig. 1.11).

While holding at the neckline, the gown is allowed to unfold completely with inner side facing the wearer (Fig. 1.12).

Slip both hands into the open armholes keeping the hands at shoulder level and away from the body. Push both hands and forearm into the sleeves of the gown but advance hands up to the proximal edge of the cuff. Do not allow hands to come out of the cuff (Figs 1.13 and 1.14). Ungloved hand should not touch the front of the gown.

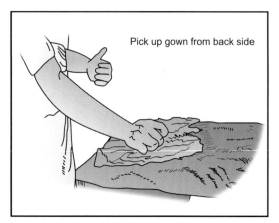

Fig. 1.11: Pick up the gown from inner side near neck

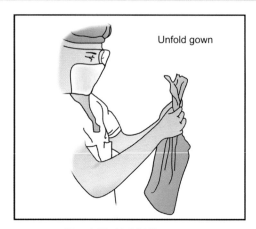

Fig. 1.12: Unfold the gown

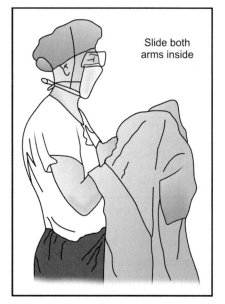

Fig. 1.13: Slide hands and arms in to the sleeves

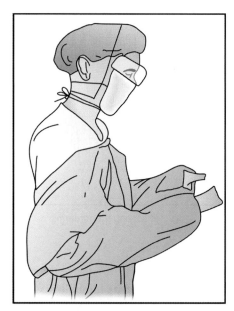

Fig. 1.14: Slide the arms into sleeves the full distance but without protruding fingers from the cuffs

The gown is secured at the back by the circulating staff (Figs 1.15 to 1.16).

Rules to observe while wearing sterile gowns and gloves.

1. Do not drop hands below the level of the umbilicus or below the sterile working area.
2. Never place hands behind the back.
3. Gloved hands must be kept within full view at all times.
4. Do not tuck gloved hands under the arm pits, as axillary region is considered contaminated.
5. Never touch an un-sterile area with gloved hands.

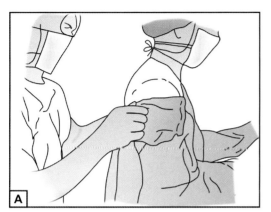

Figs 1.15A and B: Adjustment of the gown over the shoulder

Gloving

Closed gloving is the technique of choice because gloves are handled through the fabric of the gown sleeves, thereby preventing bare hands from coming into contact with the outside of the glove.

Gloving Technique

1. Hands are advanced into the sleeves of the gown till the cuff is reached.
2. The glove packet is opened in such a way that the right glove faces the right hand.
3. Pick up the left glove by its folded cuff edge with a sleeve covered right hand (Fig. 1.17).
4. Place the glove on the opposite gown sleeve, palm down, with the glove fingers pointing towards shoulder (Figs 1.18 to 1.20). The palm of the hand inside the gown sleeve must be facing upwards towards the palm of the glove. Hold the bottom rolled edge of the glove with thumb and index finger (Fig. 1.21).
5. Grasp the uppermost edge of the glove's cuff with the opposite hand and stretch the cuff of the glove over the hand. Put left hand covered with gown sleeve into glove's cuff (Fig. 1.22). Advance your finger out of the gown sleeve inside the cuff of the glove and adjust them into the respective finger stalk. Adjust the glove

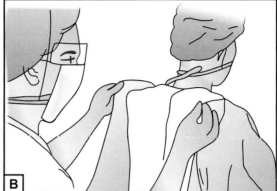

Fig. 1.16: Circulating staff secures the gown at the neck

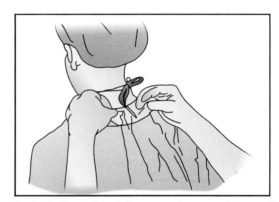

Fig. 1.17: Picking up a glove by its folded cuff edge with a sleeve-covered hand

over the gown sleeve with right hand covered with gown sleeve (Fig. 1.23).
6. Don right glove in a similar manner.

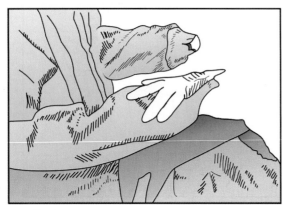

Fig. 1.18: Place the glove on the opposite sleeve

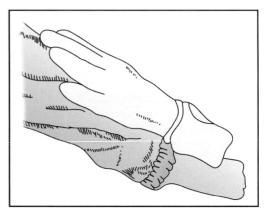

Fig. 1.19: Place the glove on the opposite sleeve (Left glove on right sleeve)

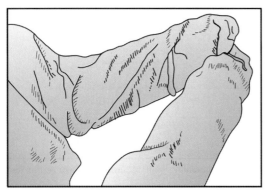

Fig. 1.20: Glove should be placed in such a way that the rolled edge of the gloved cuff is at the junction of gown cuff and sleeve

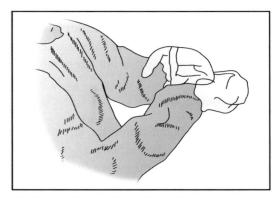

Fig. 1.21: Hold the bottom rolled edge of the glove with thumb and index finger

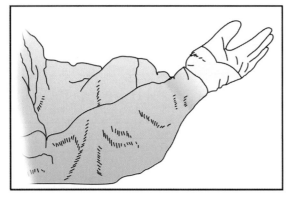

Fig. 1.22: Stretching the glove cuff over the hand

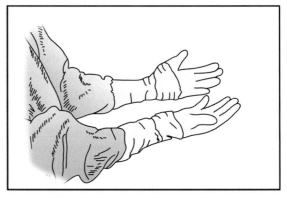

Fig. 1.23: Pulling the glove on to the hand

Final Tie of the Gown (After Donning Gloves)

If the gown is cotton, the waist tie can only be passed around behind the gowned person by a scrubbed and gowned member of staff, to maintain sterility.

If the gown is a paper disposable one, then a disposable tab attached to the waist tie can be handed to a non-scrubbed member of staff to be passed around the waist. The disposable tab is then discarded (Figs 1.24 to 1.28).

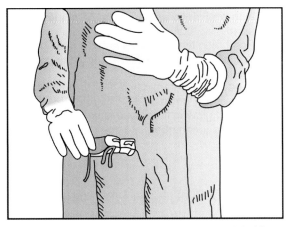

Fig. 1.24: Scrubbed person holds the paper tab holding belt and belt tie

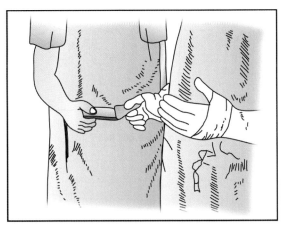

Fig. 1.25: Paper tab holding belt passed to circulating staff

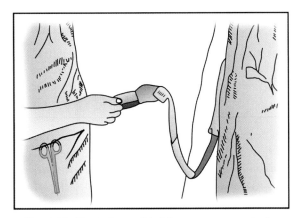

Fig. 1.26: Circulating staff holding paper comes to the side of the scrubbed person

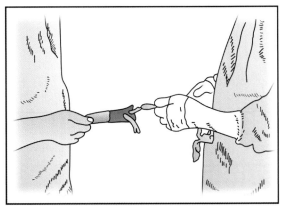

Fig. 1.27: Scrubbed person hold the belt without touching the paper tab and pull on the belt

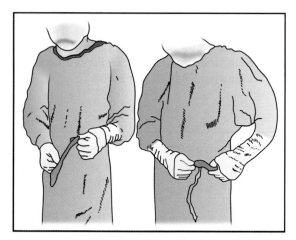

Fig. 1.28: Scrubbed person will take hold of the belt tie and tie the belt to it

KEY POINTS

1. The purpose of scrubbing is to reduce number of organisms on skin so that the risk to the patient is less if gloves become perforated during surgery.
2. One can scrub with antiseptic solution or with soap.
3. Recommended scrubbing time is 2 minutes with antiseptic solution and 5 minutes with soap.
4. Scrubbing time does not include rinsing time.
5. While wearing a gown one should touch only the inside of the gown.
6. A gown is contaminated if one touches outside of the gown.
7. Closed gloving technique is better than open gloving technique.

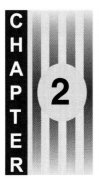

Knots are used in surgery for approximation of tissues or for ligation of blood vessels. More than 1400 knots have been described in Encyclopedias of knots, but only a few are used in surgery. The type of surgical knot used depends upon the material used, location, depth of the incision and the amount of stress placed upon the wound.

Multifilament sutures are easier to tie than monofilament sutures, because they have a high coefficient of friction and the knots remain in position as they are laid down, in comparison to the monofilament variety which have a low coefficient of friction, resulting in the knot having a tendency to loosen. Monofilament sutures have memory, and they tend to return to their resting shape. While tying knots, surgeons must work slowly and meticulously, as undue speed in knot tying may result in a poor tie, and slippage.

Safe Principals of Knot Tying

1. The completed knot must be firm to avoid slipping.
2. Knot must be as small as possible and ends should be cut short.
3. Whilst tying a knot, friction between strands must be avoided as this can weaken the suture.
4. Avoid excessive tension to the suture while applying knot.
5. Final tension on the final throw should be as nearly horizontal as possible.
6. Care should be taken to avoid damage to the suture material when handling it.

7. Tension should be maintained on the knot after the first loop has been tied to avoid loosening of the throw.
8. Extra ties do not add to the strength of a properly tied and squared knot but only add to the bulk.

Methods of Knot Tying

1. Hand tied knot
2. Instrument tied knot
3. Endoscopic knot tying

A hand tied knot can be:
1. Granny knot
2. Square knot or reef knot
3. Surgeon's knot
4. Reverse surgeon's knot
5. Double-double knot

A hand tied knot can be either by one hand or by two hands.

The Importance of Knot Tying

The knot is the weakest link in a tied surgical suture. The consequences of suboptimal and faulty knot construction may be disastrous. For example, massive hemorrhage may result from a poorly tied knot on a large artery. Knot disruption may also lead to wound dehiscence or incisional hernia.

It is important to understand the mechanical performance of a united and knotted suture, and an important consideration in a suture's mechanical performance includes knot breakage and knot slippage.

Components of a Knotted Suture Loop

A tied suture has three components:
1. The loop created by a knot maintains approximation of the divided wound edge.
2. A knot is composed of a number of throws snagged against each other. A throw is a wrapping or weaving of two strands.
3. Ears act as insurance that the loop will not become untied because of knot slippage.

Each throw within a knot can be either a single or double throw. A single throw is formed by wrapping the two strands around each other so that the rotation of the wrap is 360°.

In a double throw, the free end of the strand is passed twice instead of once around the other strand. The rotation of this double wrap throw is 720°.

Square knot: When the right ear and the loop of the two throws exit on the same side of the knot or parallel to each other.

Granny knot: When the right ear and loop exit or cross different sides of the knot.

Surgeon's knot: It comprise of initial double throw followed by a single throw.

Reverse surgeon's knot: It comprise of initial double throw followed by a single throw and then followed by a double-wrap throw.

Double-double knot: It consists of two double throws.

One handed square knot technique: It can be tied using either hand.

This type of knot is employed if using a suture with a needle attached to it. After passing the needle through tissue, the thread is pulled until the end of the suture attached to the needle is long. One handed tying of a knot uses two types of throws, i.e. index finger throw and middle finger throw. If the short end is away from the operator then the index finger throw is used. If the short end is towards the operator, the middle finger throw is used. If the short end is towards the right hand side of operator, then one can use either index finger throw by left hand or middle finger throw by right hand. If the short end is towards the left side of operator, then one can use middle finger by left hand or index finger throw by right. Crossing of hands at the end of each throw is important. It means the short end is away from the operator, it should come towards the operator at the end of throw. Crossing of hands is also known as squaring of the knot and is important, so that the knot does not become an unsafe slip knot.

1. Hold the short end of suture between the thumb and ring finger of the left hand with the loop over the extended index finger. Hold the remainder of the suture material with the right hand. Abduct the left index finger, so that short end of suture forms a loop (Fig. 2.1).
2. Bring the suture held in right hand near loop of short end held in left hand, by moving right hand away from you (Fig. 2.2).
3. Bring the index finger of left hand in front of thread held between left thumb and ring finger (Fig. 2.3).
4. Pronate the left hand so that the left index finger brings the thread held between left thumb and ring finger inside the loop.
5. Pull the thread out of loop by grasping it between left index and middle finger and complete the throw by bringing left hand towards you and right hand away from you (Fig. 2.4).
6. Continue to hold the short end of the suture in left hand between thumb and index finger. Flex and abduct left index finger so that it lies at right angle to remaining left hand fingers (Fig. 2.5).
7. Bring the thread held in the right hand across the left middle finger towards the operator to cross the left handed thread (Fig. 2.6).

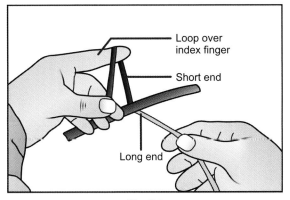

Loop over
index finger

Short end

Long end

Fig. 2.1

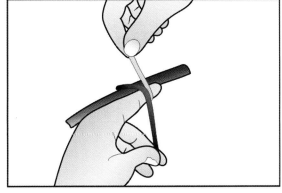

Fig. 2.2

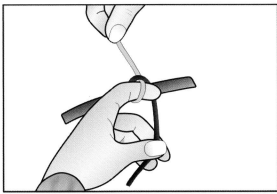

Fig. 2.3

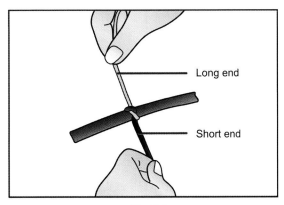

Long end

Short end

Fig. 2.4

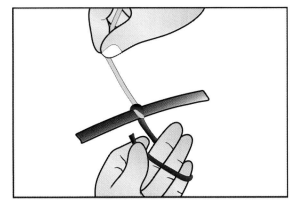

Fig. 2.5

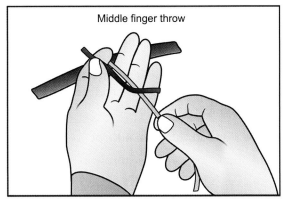

Middle finger throw

Fig. 2.6

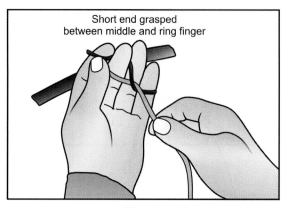

Fig. 2.7

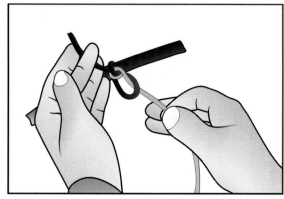

Fig. 2.8

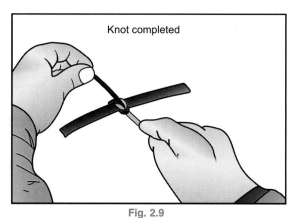

Fig. 2.9

Figs 2.1 to 2.9: Various steps of single handed reef knot

8. Use middle finger of left hand to bring short end under the right handed strand of suture. (Figs 2.7 to 2.11).
9. Grasp the short end between left middle and ring finger and bring short end away from you and tightened the knot.

Single Handed Surgeon's Knot

In this knot there is double throw in the first half knot. To create this knot the short end is drawn twice through the loop made over index before pulling the short end towards operator. Knot is completed by making a middle finger throw.

Double Handed Reef Knot

A double handed reef knot is used if there is a free suture without needle attached to it. So instead of the short end and long end, there will be two equal ends. One end away from operator and one end towards operator.

1. End away from operator is placed over extended index finger of left hand and held in palm of left hand, keeping left thumb free. Other end is held in right hand (Fig. 2.11).
2. End held in right hand is brought between left thumb and index finger (Fig. 2.12).

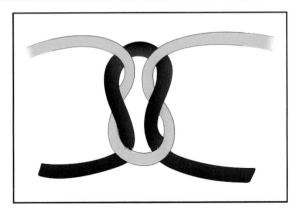

Fig. 2.10A: Cross-section of completed reef knot

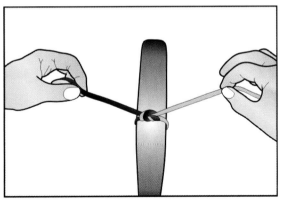

Fig. 2.10B: Completed reef knot final appearance

3. Left hand is turned inwards by pronation and thumb is brought under the end over left index finger to form the first loop (Fig. 2.13).

4. End held in right hand is crossed over the loop on left thumb and held between thumb and index finger of left hand (Fig. 2.14).

5. Right hand releases the end held by it. Left hand still holding the other end between index finger and thumb is supinated and brings the other end through the loop formed over left index finger (Fig. 2.15).

6. Other end released by left hand and grasped by right hand.

7. First half knot completed by applying horizontal tension and crossing hands (Fig. 2.16).

8. Left hand supinated and loop formed over left thumb (Fig. 2.17).

9. End held in right hand is brought in between left thumb and index finger and is crossed over the loop formed on thumb by end held in left hand.

10. Left hand supinated (Fig. 2.18).

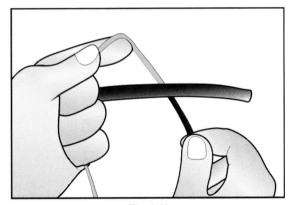

Fig. 2.11

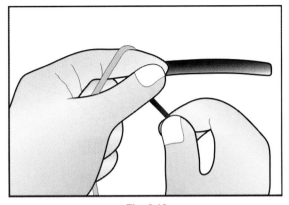

Fig. 2.12

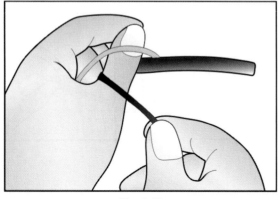

Fig. 2.13

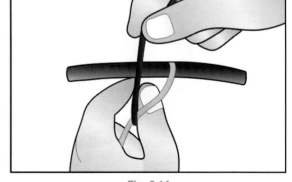

Fig. 2.14

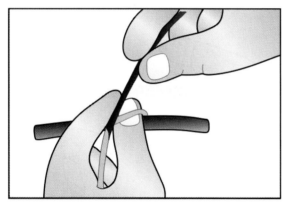

Fig. 2.15

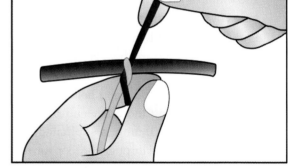

Fig. 2.16

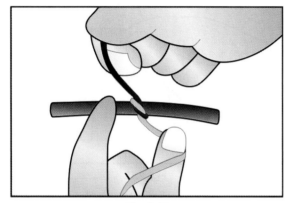

Fig. 2.17

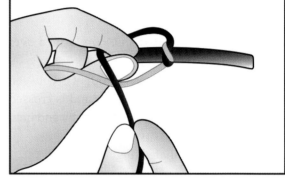

Fig. 2.18

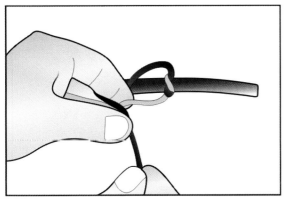

Fig. 2.19

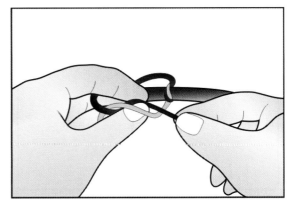

Fig. 2.20

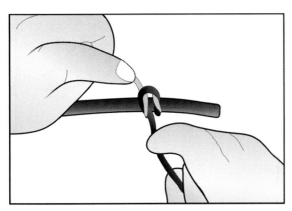

Fig. 2.21

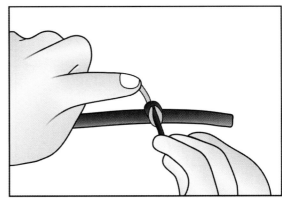

Fig. 2.22

Figs 2.11 to 2.22: Various steps of two hand tied reef knot

11. End held in the right hand is now held between left thumb and index fingers (Fig. 2.19).
12. Left hand is pronated and rotated inwards thus carrying the other end through the loop formed over left thumb (Fig. 2.20).
13. Right sided end is regrasped between right thumb and index finger.
14. Second half knot completed by applying horizontal tension across two ends (Figs 2.20 to 2.22).

15. Final tension on the final throw should be as nearly horizontal as possible.

Surgeon's Knot by Two Hands (Figs 2.23 to 2.33)

This differs from two handed square knot in the first half. Other end held in right hand is passed through the loop formed over left index finger twice, before pulling the two ends in opposite direction in horizontal plane.

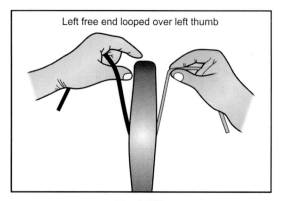

Left free end looped over left thumb

Fig. 2.23A

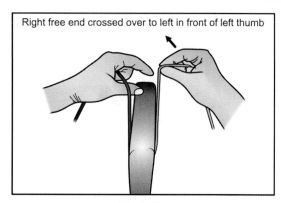

Right free end crossed over to left in front of left thumb

Fig. 2.23B

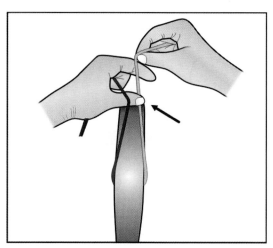

Fig. 2.24A

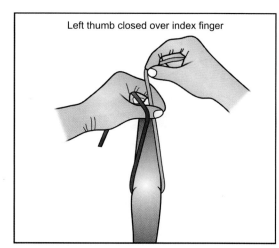

Left thumb closed over index finger

Fig. 2.24B

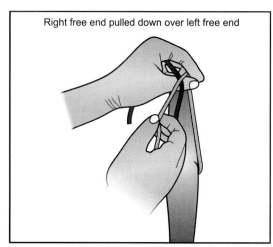

Right free end pulled down over left free end

Fig. 2.25A

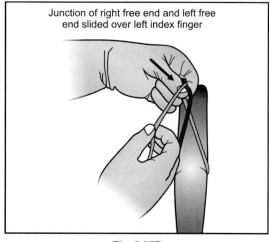

Junction of right free end and left free end slided over left index finger

Fig. 2.25B

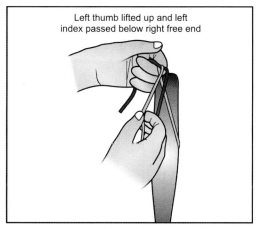

Left thumb lifted up and left
index passed below right free end

Fig. 2.26A

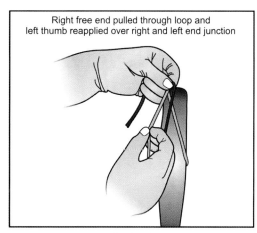

Right free end pulled through loop and
left thumb reapplied over right and left end junction

Fig. 2.26B

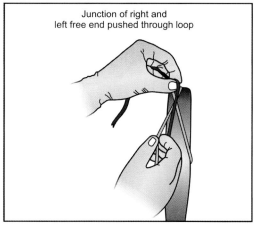

Junction of right and
left free end pushed through loop

Fig. 2.27A

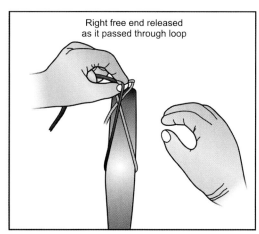

Right free end released
as it passed through loop

Fig. 2.27B

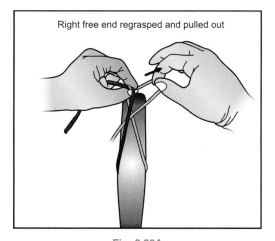

Right free end regrasped and pulled out

Fig. 2.28A

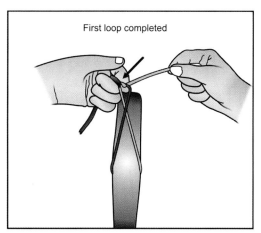

First loop completed

Fig. 2.28B

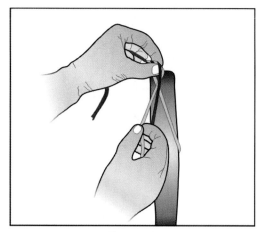

Fig. 2.29A

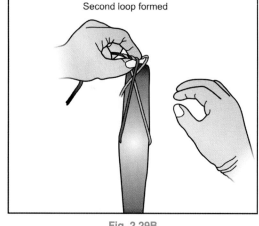

Second loop formed

Fig. 2.29B

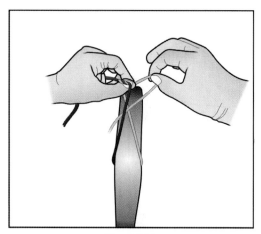

Fig. 2.30A

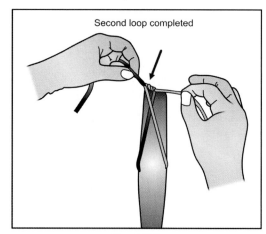

Second loop completed

Fig. 2.30B

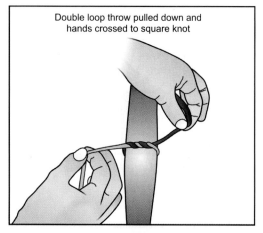

Double loop throw pulled down and
hands crossed to square knot

Fig. 2.31A

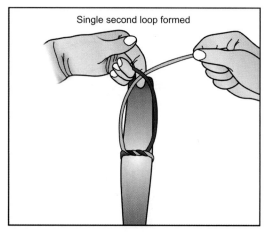

Single second loop formed

Fig. 2.31B

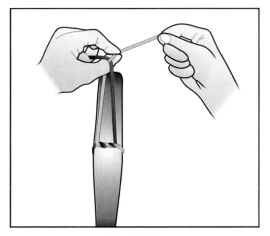

Fig. 2.32A

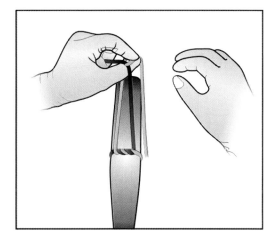

Fig. 2.32B

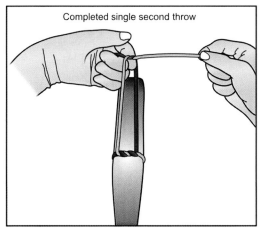

Completed single second throw

Fig. 2.33A

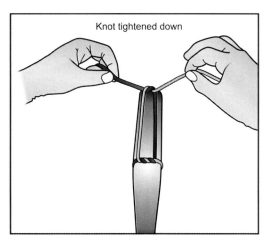

Knot tightened down

Fig. 2.33B

Figs 2.23 to 2.33: Various steps of two hand tied surgeon's knot

Instrument tied knot: Instrument tie is useful when one or both ends of the suture material are short.

Steps of instrument tied surgeon's knot:

1. Short end lies freely away from the operator and long end held between thumb and index finger of left hand, thus creating an English letter 'V' between short end and long end (Fig. 2.34).
2. Place needle holder inside 'V' and make two loops over the needle holder by the long end (Fig. 2.35).
3. Needle holder in right hand grasps the short end of the thread (Fig. 2.36).
4. First half of the knot completed by pulling needle holder towards operator side thus bringing the short end towards the operator (Fig. 2.37).
5. Long end again held between left thumb and index.
6. Needle holder held in right hand again placed in the 'V' formed by long end and short end (Fig. 2.38).

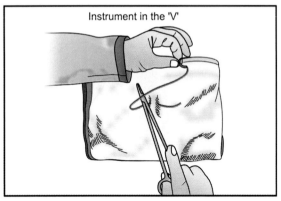

Instrument in the 'V'

Fig. 2.34

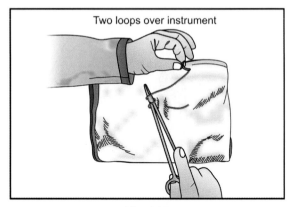

Two loops over instrument

Fig. 2.35

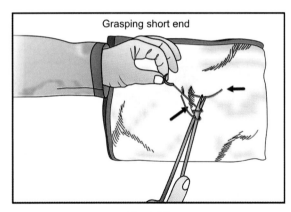

Grasping short end

Fig. 2.36

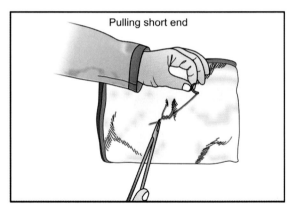

Pulling short end

Fig. 2.37

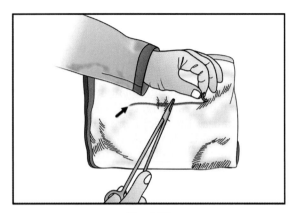

Fig. 2.38

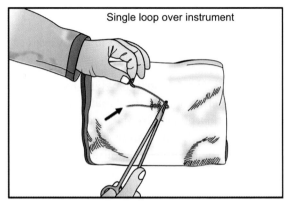

Single loop over instrument

Fig. 2.39

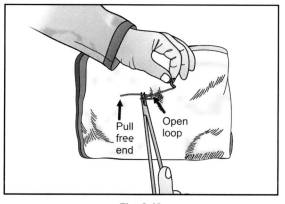

Fig. 2.40

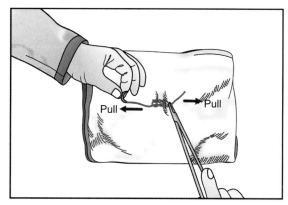

Fig. 2.41

Figs 2.34 to 2.41: Various steps of instrument tied surgeon's knot

7. Loop formed over needle holder by long end (Fig. 2.39).
8. Short end is pulled through loop, away from operator and long end towards operator (Fig. 2.40).
9. Knot is completed by horizontal tension applied by left hand holding long end and right hand holding short end in needle holder. Tension should be as nearly horizontal as possible (Fig. 2.41).

Endo Knotting

Both intracorporeal and extracorporeal suturing and knot tying techniques are used in laparoscopic surgery.

Extracorporeal Knot Tying

A Roeder's knot is widely used in laparoscopic surgery for extracorporeal tying. Commercially available pre-tied loops also have a Roeder's knot. Chromic catgut or vicryl is generally used for making a pre tied loop because chromic catgut slips easily. A loop can be made by the surgeon. Self made loops are cheaper.

Steps in Making a Roeder's Knot

1. A loop is formed over the left index finger (Fig. 2.42).
2. Tail end of the loop is brought out of the loop making a full circle (Fig. 2.42).
3. Three full circles are thrown on the tail end of the loop (Fig. 2.43).
4. Tie is closed by encircling both limbs of the loop to complete the final full circle (Figs 2.44 and 2.45).

Indications for Loop Application

1. For ligation of pedicles.
2. For ligation of the base of the appendix.
3. In case of a wider cystic duct when appropriate size clip is not applicable.
4. For control of bleeding vessels.
5. For ligation of a hernial sac in indirect hernia.

Intracorporeal Suturing

Pre-requisite for making an intracorporeal knot:
1. Suture should be neither too long nor too short. 8-10 cm length of sutures is adequate for one stitch and additional 3 cm for each extra stitch.

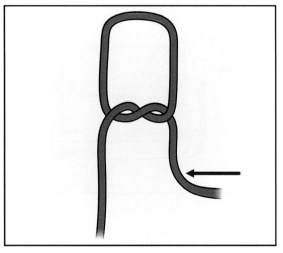

Fig. 2.42

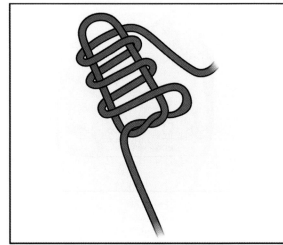

Fig. 2.43

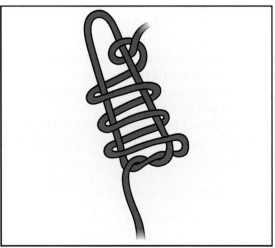

Fig. 2.44

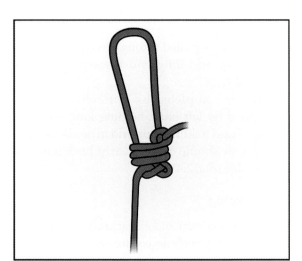

Fig. 2.45

Figs 2.42 to 2.45: Various steps of tying Roeder's knot

2. A curved or "ski" needle is used for endo-suturing. Needle is loaded reversely into reducing sleeve.
3. Left hand forceps should be atraumatic tissue grasping forceps.
4. Needle should be grasped by the needle holder at a right angle to its jaws. Needle tips with high tapering ratio or a "taper cut" tip will penetrate tissue layers more readily.
5. There should be an angle of 60-70° between right and left hand instrument.
6. Ports should be placed in such a way that principal of triangulation is followed
7. Vicryl or PDS is ideal for endosuturing.

Technique of Square and Surgeon's Knot

Over Hand Flat Knot

1. Create a C loop held in the horizontal plane.
2. Thread should lie flat against the tissue.
3. Right instrument holds the long tail and left instrument is placed over the loop (Fig. 2.46).
4. The short tail should be long enough to avoid accidentally pulling out but not so long that its end is hidden.
5. Use a large loop to allow sufficient room for movement of both instruments.
6. Use the right instrument to wrap the long tail around the stationary tip of the left instrument (Fig. 2.47).
7. Both instruments move towards the short tail.
8. Left instrument is used to grasp the tip of the short tail end and pulled out of the wrap to the right completing first flat knot (Fig. 2.48).
9. Pull the short tail through the loop and adjust it so that there is an equal length left. Pull the two instruments in opposite directions.

10. Left instrument then drops the short tail and right instrument keeps its grasp on the long tail (Fig. 2.49).

Second Opposing Flat Knot

1. Right instrument is brought to the left side of the field and rotated clockwise 180°.
2. Right instrument transfers the long tail to the left instrument thus creating a reverse C loop
3. Right instrument is placed over the reversed C loop and the left instrument wraps the thread around right instrument (Fig. 2.50).
4. Tips of both instruments are moved together in unison towards the short tail which is grasped with the right instrument.
5. Pull the short tail through the loop and then both tails in opposite directions parallel to the stitch with equal tension to configure the knot (Fig. 2.50).

Slip Knot Conversion for the Square Knot (Sezabo Technique)

This is essential to tighten the first half knot to provide adequate grip (Figs 2.51 to 2.53).

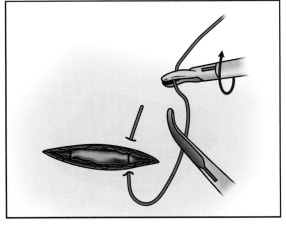

Fig. 2.46A

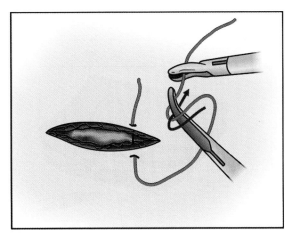

Fig. 2.46B

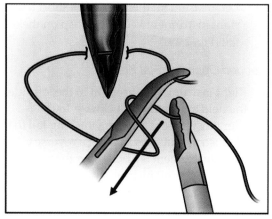

Fig. 2.47

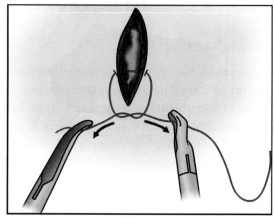

Fig. 2.48

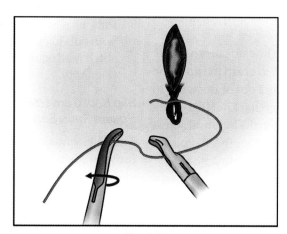

Fig. 2.49

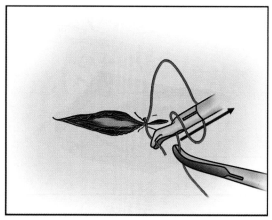

Fig. 2.50A

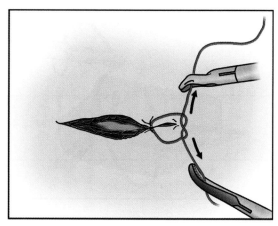

Fig. 2.50B

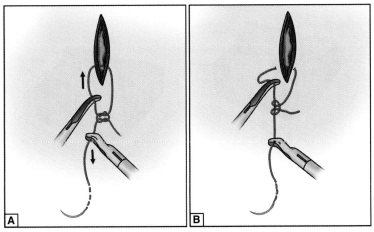

Figs 2.51A and B

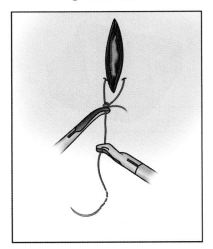

Fig. 2.52

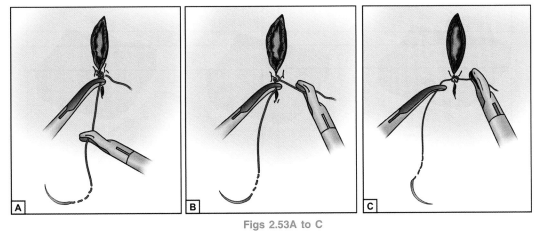

Figs 2.53A to C

Figs 2.46 to 2.53: Various steps of intracarporeal knotting

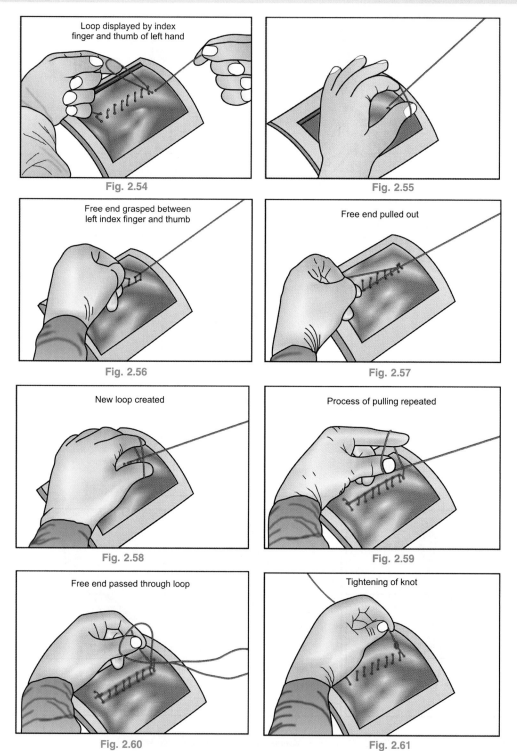

Figs 2.54 to 2.61: Various steps of Aberdeen knot tying

1. Both instruments grasp the loop on same side one below the knot and one above the knot
2. Both instruments pull in opposite directions until a snapping or popping sensation can be felt. Conversion is easier in monofilament suture.
3. Pushing the slip knot. The right instrument maintains its grasp on the tail and pulls it tightly. Left instrument pushes the knot closer to the tissue by sliding on this tail.
4. Clinch down the slip knot till tissue edges have been approximated.
5. Reconvert slip knot to square knot by pulling ends in opposite directions.

The Aberdeen Knot (Figs 2.54 to 2.61)

This knot is applied while finishing a continuous suture, when left with a loop and a free end. To tie this knot, loop is displayed between the index finger and thumb of left hand free end is grasped between the index finger and thumb of the left hand through the loop and by pulling it through and releasing the right hand thread, old loop is eliminated. New loop is formed again between left index finger and thumb and right hand thread is pulled again. Whole process is repeated 6-7 times using 'sea saw' movement.

Finally the free end is passed through the loop and tightened down.

KEY POINTS

1. Knots are used for approximation of tissues and ligation of blood vessels.
2. Multifilament sutures are easier to tie than monofilament suture and give a more secure knot.
3. Surgeon's knot or square knot should be used as far as possible.
4. Granny knot should not be used as it is not a safe knot.
5. Whatever type of knot is used the hands should cross after one throw to lock it and make it safe.

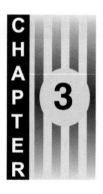

Wound Closure Techniques

The majority of lacerations can be repaired by primary wound closure. Primary wound closure has the following advantages:

1. Brings wound edges together neatly and evenly
2. Stops bleeding
3. Preserves function of the tissue
4. Prevents infection
5. Restores cosmetic appearance
6. Promotes rapid healing
7. Decreases patient discomfort

Time of Wound Closure

There seems to be a direct relationship between the time of wound closure and risk of infection. Wounds of the face and scalp can be closed by primary closure up to 72 hours after injury without increasing the risk of infection because of high vascularity. In other areas there is no significant time related difference in infection rates for wounds closed within 18 hours.

Increased Risk of Infection

There is a high incidence of wound infection after laceration repair in the following conditions:

1. Diabetes mellitus
2. Obesity
3. Malnourishment
4. Immune suppressed state
5. Patient on steroids or chemotherapeutic agents
6. Crush injuries leading to devitalized tissue
7. Contaminated wounds with foreign bodies

Wound that have been grossly contaminated, infected or have come to medical attention late are allowed to heal by secondary intention or a delayed primary closure is performed after dealing with infection.

Wound Closure Techniques

There are four main options for wound closure available. These include:

1. Sutures—These are the commonest method used
2. Tissue adhesives
3. Staples
4. Surgical tapes

Suturing of Lacerations

Suturing of lacerations is generally performed under local anesthesia except in the following situations which may require general anesthesia.

1. Large lacerations where the requirement of local anesthesia will exceed the toxic dose.
2. Severe contamination requiring extensive cleaning or removal of foreign body or extensive debridement.
3. Open fractures, tendon, nerve or major blood vessel injury.
4. Complex structures requiring meticulous repair, e.g. eyelid.

Equipment Required for Wound Suturing

1. Universal precautions kit.
2. Suturing tray containing needle holder, toothed forceps, suture scissors.

3. 1% or 2% lignocaine with or without adrenaline for local anesthesia.
4. 10 cc syringe and 21-25 gauge needle for infiltrating anesthesia.
5. Appropriate suture.
6. Wound preparation and cleaning materials, e.g. povidone iodine solution, gauze pieces, normal saline.
7. Tetanus immunization serum and syringe.

Steps of Laceration Suturing

1. Wound assessment.
2. Wound preparation.
3. Wound closure.
4. Tetanus prophylaxis.

Wound Assessment

1. Establish approximate time of injury. After four hours, wound should be scrubbed to remove the protein coagulum.
2. Determine exact mechanism of injury which can point towards underlying fracture, retained foreign body, tendon or nerve injury or wound contamination.
3. Ask about tetanus immunization status.
4. Test for distal sensory and motor function to rule out nerve and tendon injuries.
5. Consider imaging studies if there is a radiopaque retained foreign body such as glass.

Wound Preparation

Hair removal may be required for more precise wound closure. However, shaving might introduce infection. Clipping the hairs may be a better approach than shaving. Eye brows are not usually trimmed or shaved because the hair may regrow in abnormal patterns.
1. Wound cleaning is done either by direct scrubbing or irrigation of the tissue. Vigorous scrubbing may lead to tissue damage which may lead to infection.
2. Wound irrigation is another method of wound preparation. Wound irrigation can be either by continuous or pulsatile irrigation. Continuous high pressure irrigation by syringe significantly reduces bacterial count, and is particularly useful in dense contaminated tissue with limited vascularity such as a lower extremity wound. Irrigation pressures between 5 and 8 psi are appropriate and can be readily obtained with a 30-60 ml syringe and a 19 gauge needle. High pressure irrigation is contraindicated in a well vascularised location with delicate soft tissue such as eye lid, because it can lead to tissue damage in these areas with an increase in infection rate.

A variety of solutions, e.g. detergents, hydrogen peroxide and concentrated betadine have been used to irrigate wounds, but these are no longer recommended because of damaging effects on tissues. Normal saline is the irrigation solution of choice because it does not damage tissue; it is widely available and inexpensive. 100cc of saline is used for each cm of wound.

If using plain lignocaine for local anesthesia it should be buffered by adding 1 ml of sodium bicarbonate to 9 ml of lignocaine to reduce pain of injection. Inject slowly, subdermally, beginning inside the cut margin of the wound. Avoid piercing intact skin. Maximum dose of lignocaine is 4 mg/kg.

Wound Suturing

Face

Use 4-0 or 5-0 monofilament suture on a cutting needle, either absorbable or a non-absorbable can be used. Type of stitch used is either simple interrupted or sub-cuticular. Layered closure may be needed if deep, with 3-0 or 4-0 vicryl to muscle. Sutures are removed in 5 days.

Scalp

2-0 or 3-0 non-absorbable monofilament suture on a cutting needle is used for suturing. Sutures are removed in 10 days.

Lip

4-0 or 5-0 synthetic absorbable suture on tapercut needle is used for the deeper layers. 3-0 synthetic monofilament on cutting needle is used for skin. Simple interrupted sutures are applied for deeper layers and for skin.

Oral Cavity

4-0 absorbable gut or synthetic absorbable on tapercut needle is used for suturing employing a mattress technique.

Types of Sutures

Simple Interrupted Suture

This is the most common suture employed for closure of lacerations. A fine smooth non absorbable suture, e.g. Nylon or polypropylene is used for this because it causes much less tissue reaction than silk. Cutting needles are used for applying this suture. The needle should pass at a right angle to the incision line and should pass through the whole thickness of the wound (Fig. 3.1). If the depth of the incised wound is 'X' then needle should pass at a distance of one 'X' from the cut margin of wound and come out at a distance of 'X' from the other margin of the wound, so that the distance between entry and exit point of suture in skin is '2X' (Fig. 3.2). This rule does not apply to deep wounds more than 1 cm deep, where layered closure is required.

Sutures should be tied with a tension just enough to approximate the edges without causing constriction. If sutures are tied too tightly they will cause ischemia, delay healing and increase

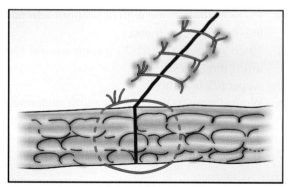

Fig. 3.1: Suture should be placed at right angle to the wound edge and should traverse whole thickness of wound

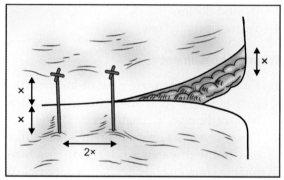

Fig. 3.2: Bite should be at a distance of X from the wound margin and come out at a distance of X from the opposite wound margin. X is the thickness of wound. Distance between two suture should be '2X'

scarring. Knots should be placed laterally away from the wound. The next stitch should be placed at a distance of '2X' from the previous stitch (Fig. 3.2) When cutting sutures, the length of left out tails from knot should be just less than 1 cm. If the tails are too long they will entangle with the next stitch, and if tails are left too short, knot slippage is a danger of knot slippage and there will be difficulty in suture removal. Sutures are generally removed around 7th day except in the face where they are removed on 5th day. Below the knee and on the back, sutures are left for 10-14 days to prevent wound dehiscence.

Vertical Mattress Suture (Fig. 3.3)

This suture is commonly used for closing surgical wounds. It is useful if there is excess skin or loose subcutaneous fat. There are two entry and two exit points. All points lie in the same line. Firstly, the needle enters the skin at a right angle at a distance from the wound margin of 'X'(depth of wound) or 1 cm if a wound is deep and a layered closure has been performed. It traverses the whole thickness of the wound, and the needle comes out from the other side of the wound at a distance of 'X' or 1 cm. Secondly, the direction of needle is reversed. The needle is placed close to the margin of the wound, traversing epidermis only in such a manner that all four points lie in same line, and the skin edges are everted. The knot is tied to one side (Figs 3.2 and 3.4).

Horizontal Mattress Suture (Figs 3.6 and 3.7)

This is another eversion suture, and may be used where the skin is thick, for example on the sole of

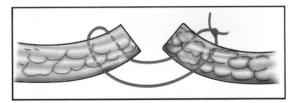

Fig. 3.5: Eversion of skin margin by vertical mattress suture

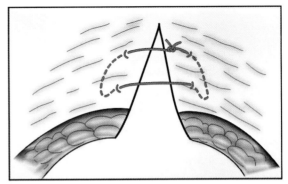

Fig. 3.6: Horizontal mattress suture

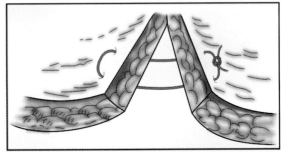

Fig. 3.7: Eversion of skin margin by horizontal mattress suture

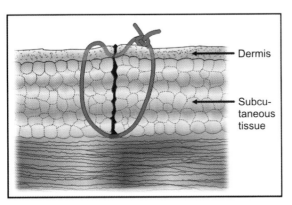

Dermis

Subcutaneous tissue

Fig. 3.3: Method of taking vertical mattress suture

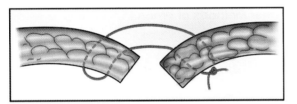

Fig. 3.4: Inversion of skin edges by vertical mattress suture

the foot. There are again two entry and two exit points. Firstly, the needle is placed 4 to 8 mm from the wound edge. It then passes through to the opposite wound edge, where it exits the skin. The needle is reversed in the needle holder, and inserted into the same skin edge 4 to 8 mm further down the wound , and passed from this side back to the other side of the wound. The needle exits the skin about 4 to 8 mm down the original wound edge from the initial insertion site.

This suture is shown in Figures 3.6 and 3.7. The main problem with this suture is that skin which is caught between each horizontal bite may lose its circulation when the knot is tied. These areas of ischemia may extend up to 50% of the entire skin margin as further sutures are placed. Partial necrosis of the skin margin is therefore quite common.

Subcuticular Suture (Fig. 3.8)

This suture gives a very fine and neat scar because approximation of skin margins is perfect. Either absorbable or non-absorbable suture can be used for this technique. For absorbable sutures, the ends are secured by means of a buried knot. For non absorbable sutures, the ends are secured by means of beads or a knot outside. Small bites are taken of the dermis on alternate sides of the wound and these are then pulled together. A continuous subcuticular suture to appose the dermal layer of the skin is a fast and cosmetically satisfactory method of skin closure. Its main advantage is that additional scarring from sutures is avoided. Its drawback is that it gives no support to the underlying tissue. Surgical gut should not be used for this suture as it produces an intense tissue reaction. If other synthetic absorbable sutures are used, knots should be placed deep and well away from the wound edge. A non-absorbable nylon or prolene is ideal. Long wounds should have intermittent bridges or external loops of suture to facilitate suture removal.

Post-suturing Management

Cover wounds that have been sutured for 1-2 days with loose protective covering. This protects from contamination until significant epithelization has occurred. After 2 days, gentle cleansing of sutured wound is acceptable. Topical application of antibiotic ointment or petroleum jelly may allow increased rate of epithelization. A moist environment also lowers infection rates and decreases scab formation.

Prophylactic antibiotics are not indicated after a simple laceration repair but should be given in cases of contamination (including animal or human bites), crush wounds, and in diabetic patients. Antibiotics are also indicated in oral lacerations, open fractures and where joints and tendons are exposed.

Suture Removal

Sutures should be cut as close as possible to the point where it emerges from the skin on the side of incision opposite the knot (Fig. 3.9A). This enables the surgeon to draw the minimal length of the exposed and possibly contaminated suture material beneath the skin and tissues. While pulling, suture traction should be towards the incision line, not away from it (Fig. 3.9B). If the suture is pulled away from the suture line, a partially healed wound might open up.

Other Methods of Wound Closure

Tissue Adhesives

These adhesives contain cyanoacrylates which are liquid monomers made by a combination of formaldehyde and cyanoacrylate. This reacts

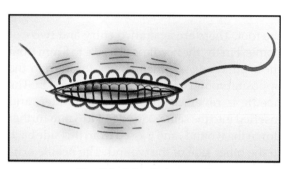

Fig. 3.8: Subcuticular suture

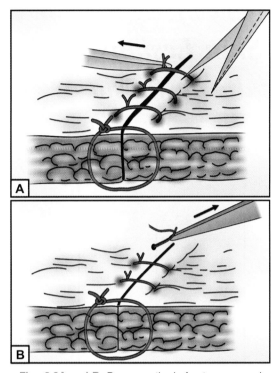

Figs 3.9A and B: Proper method of suture removal

infection rate. Staples are particularly useful for wound closure in scalp, extremity and trunk wounds. They are also commonly used on long surgical incisions.

Surgical or Adhesive Tapes (Steristrips)

These cause little skin reactivity, and are useful for very small wounds, and in children. If additional adhesive solution is required, Opsite spray is ideal, as tincture of Benzoic acid may lead to a local skin reaction or even wound infection. Tapes are not ideal for primary closure of wounds, but can be placed after suture removal and may decrease skin tension. They usually fall away in 7-10 days.

with hydroxyl ions found in water and blood, thereby causing a reaction which bonds the edges of the skin. The benefits of tissue adhesives include less pain and quick application. They are therefore potentially useful in children. Infection rates are higher with tissue adhesives. For application of tissue adhesive, skin edges should be approximated and a thin layer of adhesive evenly applied. If there is a significant tension during manual approximation, a tissue adhesive should not be used. They should not be applied over areas of high tension such as over joints or in the hand. If wrongly applied they can be easily removed with acetone, petroleum jelly or antibacterial ointment. They have some antibacterial property against gram-positive bacteria.

Staples

The benefit of skin staples includes fast application, lower rate of foreign body reaction and decreased

KEY POINTS

1. Majority of wounds should be closed primarily to have optimum cosmetic result and for preservation of function.
2. Wounds should be closed within 18 hours to avoid wound infection except for wounds of face and scalp where a delay of up to 72 hrs is acceptable.
3. Wound preparation by hair removal and irrigation by normal saline with irrigation pressure of 5-8 psi is mandatory before wound closure.
4. Povidone iodine and hydrogen peroxide should be avoided for wound irrigation as they damaging effect on tissue.
5. Simple interrupted suture should be applied as far as possible.
6. Vertical mattress should be used if there is excess of skin or loose subcutaneous fat.
7. Horizontal mattress may be useful for either eversion or inversion of a wound edge but there is a higher incidence of ischemia and necrosis of skin.
8. Subcuticular suture gives a very fine and neat scar but has the disadvantage of not providing any support to the deep tissues.

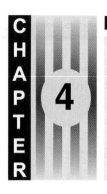

CHAPTER 4

Surgery of Common Skin Lesions Under Local Anesthesia

The indications for removal of skin lesions are as follows:

1. To rule out malignancy
2. Cosmesis
3. To improve function
4. To stop infection, bleeding, pain or irritation.

If a particular lesion is being removed for cosmetic reasons, all efforts should be made to give a neat, scar, which is less conspicuous and smaller then the original contour of the lesion.

Other options for treatment include lasers, cryosurgery, electrocautery excision, curettage or local applications of skin ointments. These should be discussed with the patient before offering excision. Accurate clinical diagnosis and dermatology input may be required. Lasers are particularly useful in arteriovenous malformations and skin lesions of neurofibromatosis, e.g. Café-au-lait spots.

Anesthesia

The majority of skin lesions can be removed under local anesthestic. This can be either used as local infiltration or as a nerve block, e.g. digital nerve block, brachial, intercostal or femoral nerve block or field block (Figs 4.1 to 4.3).

The following agents are commonly used for local anesthesia:

Lignocaine 0.5% preprepared, or prepared from 1 or 2% commercially available solutions by dilution with normal saline. Maximum dose is 4 mg/kg of body weight without adrenaline and 7 mg/kg body weight with adrenaline.

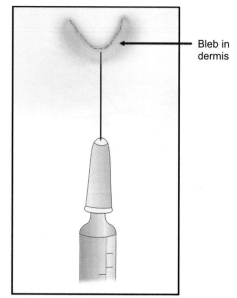

Bleb in dermis

Fig. 4.1: A bleb should be raised in the dermis by a 24 number needle before start of infiltration of local anesthesia

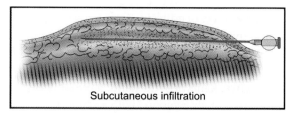

Subcutaneous infiltration

Fig. 4.2: Method of infiltration of local anesthesia in subcutaneous plane

Lignocaine 1 or 2% with 1:200,000 adrenaline gives a longer period of anesthesia because anesthetic absorption is delayed due to arteriolar

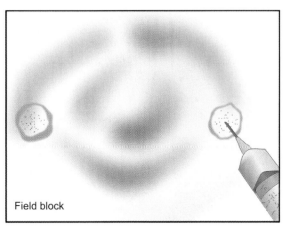

Field block

Fig. 4.3: Field block method of local anesthesia

Field Block (Fig. 4.3)

In this method the local anesthetic agent is injected into the tissues at some distance from the actual site of operation, so that a zone of anesthesia is created surrounding the operation area. The skin can be anesthetized first in the area of the block. The block itself may require a long needle. Injection is made into the subcutaneous plane, and before infiltrating the deeper planes, the syringe should be aspirated to make sure that needle has not entered into a blood vessel. During injection the needle is gradually withdrawn. The advantage of field block is that the lesion is not obscured by local swelling.

Nerve Block

Local anesthetic agent can be injected around a nerve to give anesthesia in the area which it serves. Digital nerve block is commonly employed for surgery on fingers or toes. Plain lignocaine is injected at the base of the digit on either side to block dorsal and palmar digital nerves. Injection is made in the web space on both sides of finger. The needle is pushed vertically down until it touches bone, then it is slightly withdrawn and local anesthetic is injected after confirmation by aspiration that the needle is not in a vessel. 0.5 ml of 0.5% lignocaine is sufficient on each side.

Common Skin Procedures

Excision of Sebaceous Cyst

Excision of sebaceous cyst is advised due to its tendency to grow and become infected. The cyst should be excised completely in order to avoid recurrence.

If the cyst is small and the overlying skin is healthy, a linear incision is employed. If the cyst is markedly protuberant or if the skin is thin and unhealthy or if there is an overlying punctum, an elliptical incision is used. The punctum should be in the center of the ellipse which should be equal in length to the diameter of cyst.

constriction. Delay in absorption permits use of lower doses of anesthetic. Local vasoconstriction also reduces the capillary oozing in operative field. An adrenaline containing solution should not be used in the vicinity of end arteries because vasoconstriction can endanger blood supply particularly in fingers or toes.

Bupivicaine 0.5% or 0.25% solution is available with or without adrenaline. It is a longer acting agent, but slower in onset of action, but its effect can last up to 6-8 hours, giving significantly better postoperative pain relief.

Injection of local anesthetic agent into skin can be more painful than the surgery itself. Ways to minimize this include:

Explanation of the procedure to patient with reassurance to allay anxiety.

Topical application of local anesthetic cream (a combination of lignocaine and prilocaine).

Warming the solution along with the addition of bicarbonate (0.5 ml in 9.5 ml of lignocaine) to make it less acidic.

Slow injection into subcutaneous tissue first.

Epidermal infiltration to raise a wheal with a fine (26 G) needle prior to using a large (19 G) needle for main infiltration.

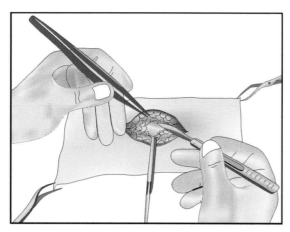

Fig. 4.4: Raising flaps for excision of sebaceous cyst

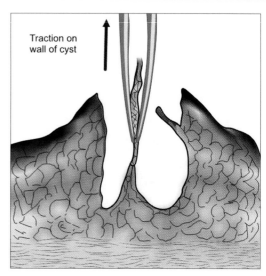

Fig. 4.5: Avulsion method of removal of sebaceous cyst

If the skin overlying the cyst is stretched, the width of the ellipse can be wider to avoid excess skin folds when closing the wound. After the skin ellipse is incised, a plane is developed between the cyst wall and the surrounding skin by sharp or blunt dissection, preferable without opening the cyst (Fig. 4.4). After dissection all around, the cyst is easily shelled out.

An alternative method is avulsion of the cyst. This is particularly suited for removal of cysts on the scalp. A comparatively small incision is required and cutaneous scarring is less. A skin flap is raised on only one side. The cyst is then deliberately opened and contents squeezed out. A pair of non-toothed dissecting forceps with one blade outside the cyst and one blade inside, cyst wall is grasped at its deepest part (Fig. 4.5) and by traction on the forceps, the entire cyst wall can be avulsed easily. The cyst wall is held at the deepest portion because the deeper part is tougher than the superficial portion and will not tear easily. The wound is sutured and a pressure dressing is applied to prevent hematoma formation in the cavity.

If the sebaceous cyst is infected, removal is deferred until the inflammation subsides. If there is abscess formation, it should be incised and pus drained. Curettage of the abscess cavity or swabbing with pure carbolic acid may prevent the cyst from reforming. Infected sebaceous cysts should not be excised as wound complication rates are high and the resulting scars are unsatisfactory. They often do not recur after incision because infection frequently destroys the lining of the cyst.

Lipoma Excison

Lipomas are excised if they are rapidly enlarging, painful, unsightly or if there is concern about malignant change. They may rarely hamper movement. For a subcutaneous lipoma excision, a skin incision is deepened through the overlying fat until the capsule of the lipoma is reached. It can be differentiated from the surrounding fat by larger fat globules, color, and a fine capsule. The lesion can often be enucleated after incision of its fine capsule, but larger lesions may need sharp dissection.

If a lipoma is adherent to the underlying muscle it should not be removed under local anesthetic as there may be deep extensions between muscle bellies, with involvement of neurovascular bundles. If a deeper lesion is suspected if the lesion is more than 5 cm in diameter, a CT or MRI scan is indicated.

Basal Cell Carcinoma (Rodent Ulcer)

Basal cell carcinoma should be excised with 2 mm of normal tissue all around on all aspects including the deeper plane. Completeness of excision should be checked by histopathology. Complete excision is associated with a recurrence rate of less than 2%. Moh has described a technique for recurrent lesions to ensure complete tumor excision. This technique essentially comprises of excision in layers with horizontal frozen section control. Radiotherapy is an alternative to surgical excision in difficult situations like penetrating lesion of eyes, nose, mouth which will require major reconstruction after complete excision.

Squamous Cell Carcinoma

These should be completely excised with 1 cm of macroscopically normal skin. Skin flaps should be extensively raised so that a still larger area of deep fascia can be excised. This tumor is sensitive to radiotherapy which may be used as an alternative or as an adjunct to operation.

Malignant Melanoma

If a malignant melanoma is suspected, the initial surgery should be carried out to excise the lesion with minimal margins to obtain the tumor depth. For a tumor excised with < 1 mm depth, a wide excision of 1 cm margin around the tumor is sufficient. If the tumor is between 1-2 mm in depth, a 1-2 cm wide margin is adequate. For tumors > 2 mm in depth, 2 cm clearance is recommended as being sufficient. The excision should be carried down to but not through deep fascia.

All patients with tumour depth of > 1 cm should be offered sentinel node biopsy at the same time as the wide excision. If the sentinel node is positive then the patient will need to have complete nodal clearance.

KEY POINTS

1. Common indications for removal of skin lesion are cosmetic, concern about malignancy, if symptomatic or if hampering the movement or function of a joint.
2. Majority of skin lesions can be removed under local anesthesia.
3. Sebaceous cyst should be removed if there is tendency to grow or if getting infected.
4. Sebaceous cyst should be removed completely to avoid recurrence.
5. Basal cell carcinoma is excised with 2 mm of normal tissue all around.
6. Squamous cell carcinoma is excised with 1 cm of normal skin.

Sutures in Surgery

Definition

The word "suture" describes any material used to ligate blood vessels and ducts, or to approximate tissues. Sutures are used to close wounds.

Use of sutures dates back to the era of the great Indian surgeon Sushruta, father of ancient Indian surgery. In 2000 BC, Egyptians and Syrians used sutures for various purposes. All sorts of materials ranging from horse hair, animal tendons, wire, silk, cotton and linen, have been used as suture materials. Some of these are still used today.

In the modern era, technical advances have brought us to a stage where specific sutures are available for a particular use.

The Ideal Suture

A single suture meeting all requirements does not exist, but an ideal suture should have the following properties:

1. It should be devoid of any allergic, carcinogenic, capillary or electrostatic action.
2. It should be easy to sterilize.
3. It should not produce any magnetic field around it, as in steel wire.
4. It should be easy to handle.
5. It should cause minimal tissue reaction.
6. It should not promote growth of bacteria around it.
7. It should hold the tissue securely throughout the phase of wound healing.
8. It should absorb with minimal tissue reaction having served its purpose.

Classification of Suture Material (Table 5.1)

Suture Size

Suture size denotes the diameter of suture material. Suture size is generally denoted by O's. As no. of "O's" in the suture size increases, diameter of suture strand decreases. Suture size is directly proportional to the tensile strength of the suture. The smaller the size of the suture, the less is the tensile strength of the suture.

Knot Tensile Strength

This is measured by the force, in pounds, which the suture strand can withstand before it breaks when knotted. Tensile strength of the tissue is measured by its ability to withstand stress. Tensile strength of the suture should always exceed the tensile strength of the tissue.

Sutures can be classified in many ways:

1. Monofilament vs. Multifilament
2. Absorbable vs. Non-absorbable
3. Natural vs. Synthetic

Working Classification of Sutures

Table 5.1	**Classification of sutures**

1. Absorbable
   i. Natural
   ii. Synthetic
2. Non-absorbable
   i. Natural
   ii. Synthetic

Natural absorbable
1. Surgical gut (plain or chromic)
2. Collagen (plain or chromic)

Natural non-absorbable
1. Surgical silk
2. Surgical Linen
3. Cotton

Synthetic absorbable
1. Polyglecaprone 25
2. Polydioxanone
3. Polyglycolic acid
4. Polyglactin 910

Synthetic non-absorbable
1. Polyamide
2. Stainless Steel
3. Polypropylene
4. Polyester (suture can be made of mono-filament or multifilament)

Monofilament vs. Multifilament

Monofilament sutures comprising a single strand of material, encounter less resistance when passing through tissue, and resist harboring organisms. This property makes them suitable for use in vascular surgery. They are easy to tie, but are delicate and easy to break. They are also more amenable to crushing or crimping.

Multifilament sutures consist of multiple filaments and strands, twisted and braided together. They may be coated for smooth passage through tissue. They have more tensile strength, pliability and flexibility. They are well suited for intestinal anastomosis.

Absorbable vs. Non-Absorbable Sutures

Sutures that undergo rapid degradation in tissue, losing their tensile strength within 60 days are known absorbable sutures. Those which maintain their tensile strength for more than 60 days are known as non-absorbable sutures. Silk loses 50 percent of its tensile strength in one year and has no strength at the end of two years. Nylon loses 25 percent of its original strength during two years. Cotton retains 30-40 percent of its original strength at the end of two years.

Absorbable Sutures

These are either derived from collagen or synthetic polymers.

Catgut Sutures

These are either derived from the submucosa of sheep intestine or from serosa of beef intestine. Collagenous tissue obtained from gut is treated with an aldehyde solution for cross linking, which gives the suture more strength and makes it resistant to enzymatic degradation. Sutures obtained in this way are known as plain gut. If plain gut is additionally treated by chromium trioxide, it is known as chromic gut. Chromic gut has more cross linkage and is more resistance to absorption. Reabsorption of gut is by enzymatic degradation, mainly by the lysosomal enzyme acid phosphatase initially, followed by leucine amino-peptidase. Collagenase also plays a significant role in degradation.

Plain gut is rapidly absorbed and maintains its tensile strength for 7-10 days and is completely absorbed in 70 days. Tensile strength of chromic gut is maintained for 14-20 days. Drawbacks of gut suture are breakage during knot tying and variation in retention of tensile strength. There is also a concern regarding transfer of prion disease.

Collagen Sutures

These are derived from homogenized Tendo Achilles of beef cattle and are 100 percent pure collagen. They are available in plain and chromic form. They are stiffer than surgical gut. Therefore handling becomes difficult in large size suture. Finer size sutures are used in eye surgery.

Fascia Lata

This is obtained from the thigh muscles of beef cattle. It used to be used for hernia repair. It is still occasionally used for surgical correction of drooping upper eye lid and for facial palsy.

Kangaroo Tendon

This is obtained from tail tendons of small Kangaroos and varies in length from 10 inches to 18 inches. It has a high tensile strength.

Synthetic Polymer Sutures

Synthetic polymer sutures available are:
1. Polyglycolic acid suture (Homomer)
2. Copolymers of glycolide and lactide (Polyglactin)
3. Poliglecaprone 25 (Monocryl)
4. Polydioxanone prepared from polyster poly.

Polyglycolic Acid Suture (Dexon, Dexon 1)

This is a homomer of polyglycolic acid. It has high tensile strength with retention of 60% strength at day 7, and 35% at day 60. This suture is completely hydrolyzed by 90-120 days. This is a multifilament suture with good handling and knot security properties. It has a high coefficient of friction, which gives rise to drag during passage through tissue.

This suture has high tissue reactivity and may potentiate infection. To minimize tissue drag, a coated form of polyglycolic acid is available. Coating is in the form of copolymer of glycoilide and Epsilon caparolactone (Dexan 1).

Polyglactin (Vicryl)*

This is a coplymer of glycolic acid and lactic acid. Polyglactin 910 consists of glycolide and lactide in the ratio of 9: 1. For every nine parts of glycolic acid there is one part of lactic acid. The lactide element is more hydrophobic than glycolic acid, and thus slows down the absorption of water by suture material, and hence the breakdown of linkage of copolymer chain is slowed down.

Vicryl comes with a coating of 50% polyglactin and 50% calcium stearate. This polyglactin coating consist of 35% glycolide and 65% lactide and is known as polyglactin 370. Calcium stearate is an absorbable organic lubricant. Coating of polyglactin 370 and calcium stearate over polyglactin 910 reduces the surface friction of the suture thus avoiding tissue drag and premature locking.

If coated polyglactin 910 is exposed to gamma irradiation, it results in a low molecular weight suture in comparison to coated polyglactin and is available as vicryl rapidae. Vicryl rapidae has 30 percent less tensile strength than coated vicryl. Coated vicryl retains 80% of post implantation tensile strength at 14 days, and 30% of tensile strength at 21 days. Absorption of coated vicryl is complete between 56 to 70 days.

Vicryl rapidae loses all its tensile strength between 10 and 12days. Vicryl rapidae is totally absorbed within 42 days.

For Knotting of Vicryl

There should be double throw in the first half knot, followed by additional two throws (Total of four throws). Ends should be cut long.

Coated vicryl sutures are suitable for use any where except in neural tissue or cardiovascular tissue. Coated vicryl rapidae suture is well suited for skin closure, episiotomy suture and closure of lacerations under plaster casts.

Please note that pharmaceutical names given in this chapter for various suture can vary from country to country

Coated vicryl plus antibacterial suture is coated vicryl with a layer of antibacterial agent Triclosan. The antibacterial agent coating offers protection against bacterial colonization of the suture.

Polydioxanone Suture (PDS and PDS II)

This monofilament synthetic suture comprises of polyester poly (p-dioxanone). It is a soft, pliable suture and provides support to tissue for 6 weeks. It elicits only slight tissue reaction. It is absorbed through hydrolysis. It retains 70% of tensile strength at 2 weeks, and 50% tensile strength at 4 weeks and 25% at 6 weeks. Absorption is minimal until about the 90th day and is essentially complete within 6 months. It has more flexibility than polyglycolic acid or polyglactin suture.

Polyglecaprone 25 (Monocryl)

This is a monofilament suture, which has superior pliability for easy handling and tying. It is a copolymer of glycolide and epsilon-caprolactone. It is composed of 75% glycolide and 25% capro-lactone and is available in undyed and dyed violet form.

This is the most pliable synthetic absorbable suture. It has a smooth surface which passes through tissue with ease. It is virtually inert, and has good tensile strength retains 50-60% of this at 7th day. All its tensile strength is lost in 21 days. It is absorbed by the mechanism of hydrolysis in 90-120 days.

Non-absorbable Sutures

Non-absorbable sutures are classified into three classes:

Class I   Silk or synthetic fibers of monofilament (twisted or braided)
Class II Cotton or linen fibers
Class III Metal wire of monofilament or multi-filament construction.

Silk

Silk sutures are non-absorbable, sterile, and non-mutagenic, consisting of natural pertinacious silk fibers called fibroin. This protein is derived from the domestic silk worm *Bombyx mori*. Silk fibers are treated to remove the naturally occurring sericin gum.

Silk sutures are braided around a core and coated with wax to reduce capillary action. They are colored black with Logwood extract. Silk, being a foreign protein, causes more tissue reaction than synthetic non-absorbable sutures. Silk induces a polymorphonuclear type of cellular reaction. Although classified as non-absorbable it behaves as a very slowly absorbing suture. It loses most of its tensile strength in about one year and usually cannot be detected in tissues after two years. Encapsulation of the silk with a fibrous capsule occurs in 14-21 days. Handling properties are good, and it knots easily and securely. Surgical silk loses tensile strength when exposed to moisture and should be used dry.

Linen

This is made from flax and is a cellulose material. It is twisted to form a fiber to make a suture. Tissue reaction is similar to silk, and handling and knotting properties are very good. It is unique in the property that it gains 10 percent in tensile strength when wet. It is still widely used for tying pedicles and as a ligature.

Cotton

It is derived from the hairs of the seeds of the cotton plant. It is twisted to form a suture. It is weak in comparison to linen, and is rarely used.

Nylon

This is composed of long chain of polyamide polymers. It has a high tensile strength and low tissue reactivity. Because of its elasticity it is well suited for abdominal and skin closure.

Nylon has a low coefficient of friction and tissue reaction is minimal. It loses 25% of tensile strength in 1 year. It has a memory and knot security is lower than that of other sutures. It is available as monofilament (Ethilon) or multi-filament strands known as Nurolen. Mono-filament nylon in a wet state is more pliable than dry nylon. Multifilament nylon sutures have more strength and elicit less tissue reaction than silk. Multifilament nylon sutures generally lose 15 to 20% of their tensile strength per year in tissue by hydroxylation.

Polyester Fiber

This comprises of untreated fibers of polyester braided into a multifilament strand. This is also known as Terylene or Dacron. It has a very high tensile strength and relatively low tissue reactivity. It retains tensile strength for an indefinite period. It has become the suture of choice for cardiovascular procedures, blood vessel anastomosis and for placement of prosthetic material. Polyester sutures have a tendency to cut through tissue and to obviate this tendency, coating of teflon or polybutylate is provided over the polyester suture. Polyester coated with polybutylate is known as Ethibond. The polybutylate coating does not increase the diameter of the suture in contrast to teflon coating and also does not flake in the tissue.

Polypropylene

This is also known as Prolene. It is a monofilament and has extremely high tensile strength which is retained for indefinite period. It has very low tissue reactivity. It can stretch up to 30% before breaking and hence is useful in situations where postoperative swelling is anticipated. Knotting is very secure because the suture deforms on knotting and allows the knot to bed down on itself. It has a low coefficient of friction and slides through tissue readily. In comparison to silk it is less thrombogenic. It is extremely smooth and does not saw through the tissues. As it does not adhere to tissue, it is useful as a "pull out" suture, e.g. subcuticular suture. Polypropylene is recommended for use where minimal suture reaction is desired, such as in contaminated and infected wounds to minimize sinus formation and suture extrusion.

Tips for Preservation of Tensile Strength of Suture

Absorbable Sutures

1. Protect them from heat and moisture. Store them at room temperature. Avoid storage in hot areas, e.g. near steam pipes, and in sterilizers.
2. Do not soak absorbable sutures.
3. To restore pliability surgical gut can be dipped in room temperature water or saline.
4. Synthetic absorbable sutures must be kept dry.

Non-Absorbable Sutures

1. *Silk*: Store silk in dry environment. Dry strands are stronger than wet strands. Wet silk looses up to 20% of its strength. Avoid kinking, nicking or instrument damage.
2. *Polyester fiber*: It is unaffected by moisture. It can be used either wet or dry. Handle it carefully to avoid abrasions, kinking, and nicking or instrument damage.
3. *Nylon*: Straighten kinks or bends by passing strands between gloved fingers a few times. Avoid kinking, nicking or instrument damage.
4. *Polypropylene*: Unaffected by moisture. It can be used wet or dry. Thread should be straightened with a gentle, steady and even pull.

Surgical Needles

Composition

Surgical needles are made up of stainless steel alloy, which is resistant to corrosion and contain a minimum of 12% chromium. When a needle is exposed to oxygen in air it forms a thin protective layer of chromium oxide.

An ideal needle should have following characteristics:

1. Made of high quality stainless steel.
2. As thin and slim as possible without compromising strength.
3. Should have a stable grasp in needle holder.
4. Should cause minimal trauma to tissue.
5. Should be able to penetrate tissue with minimal resistance.
6. Should resist bending
7. Should be resistant to breaking under a given amount of bending. In ideal needle should bend before breaking if excessive force is applied.

The Anatomy of the Needle

Components

Every surgical needle has three basic parts swage, body and point.

Swage

The swage is the site of attachment of the suture to needle. It is usually round in section. Swaged needles produce smaller holes in tissue in comparison to threaded eye needles.

Body

The body of the needle is the portion which is grasped by the needle holder during the surgical procedure. It is often square in section. The diameter of the body of the needle should be as close as possible to the diameter of the suture material to minimize bleeding and leakage. This is especially important for cardiovascular, gastro-intestinal and bladder procedures.

Point

The needle point extends from tip of the needle to the level of the maximum cross section of the body.

Types of Needle Point

Cutting needles have two opposing cutting edges.

Conventional Cutting Edge Needle

This has two opposite cutting edge and third cutting edge is on the inside of the concave curvature of the needle. The inside cutting edge produces linear cuts perpendicular and near to the incision. When the suture exerts a wound closure force, it can cut through this hole. It is primarily used for closure of skin and sternum.

Reverse Cutting Edge Needle

This has a third cutting edge on the outer convex curvature of needle. It has more strength than a conventional cutting needle. The danger of tissue cut out is much less because the hole produced by it has a wide wall of the tissue contrary to the linear cut produced by a conventional cutting needle. The wide wall against which the suture is tied resists suture cut through.

Spatula Needle

This is a side cutting needles, flat on both bottom and top, with cutting edges on the side. It is primarily used for eye surgery. It can also be used for repairing lacerations of the nail matrix. Side cutting edges split or separate the tissue without cutting them.

Taper Point Needle

This tapers to a sharp tip. It spreads the tissue without cutting it, and is used where the surgeon wants to make a smallest hole possible without cutting tissue. It is used in soft tissue, e.g. vessels, abdominal viscera and fascia which do not resist needle penetration.

Taper Cut Needle

This combines the unique features of taper point and cutting edge needles. Cutting edges extends only for a short distance from the needle tip and blends in to a round taper body. The tapercut needle is used for anastomosis of calcified and fibrotic blood vessels, to graft, and for closure of defects in oral mucosa. The penetrating point needle is a type of taper cut needle with diamond shaped point.

Blunt Point Needle

This has a taper body with a rounded, blunt point that will not cut through tissue. It is used for suturing the liver and kidney, and also to prevent needlestick injury in patients with HIV, or Hepatitis B/C infection.

Types of Needles According to Shape

1. *Straight needle*: This can be used for suturing easily accessible tissue, where direct finger-held manipulation can easily be performed (Fig. 5.1).
2. The Keith needle is a straight cutting needle for skin closure of abdominal wounds, for arthroscopic suturing of the meniscus in the knee. Bunnell (BN) This needle is used for tendon repair.
3. The half curved needle or "Ski" needle for laparoscopic anastomoses (Fig. 5.1).
4. *Curved needle*: These needles have predictable needle turn out from tissue. They require less space for maneuvering than a straight needle but require a needle holder for manipulation. The curvature of the needle may be 1/4, 3/8, 1/2, or 5/8 of a full circle. 3/8 circle is used for large superficial wounds. The curve of the needle can be manipulated with slight pronation but then has a larger arc of manipu-lation, so is not suitable in a deep body cavity or restricted area.

   1/2 circle needle is used in a confined space. 5/8 circle needle is used for hemorrhoidectomy, in the nasal cavity, oral cavity and pelvis (Fig. 5.1).

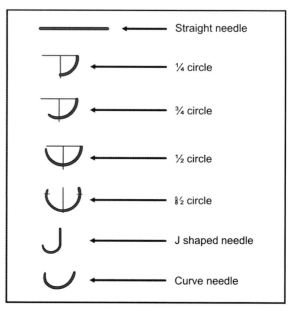

Fig. 5.1: Different shapes of surgical needles

KEY POINTS

1. Ideal sutures having all desirable properties do not exist.
2. One should choose a suture carefully keeping in mind the type of operation being performed.
3. Tensile strength of suture and ease of knotting is an important aspect to be considered while selecting suture material.
4. If selecting a non-absorbable suture one should choose a suture which maintains its tensile strength for 90-120 days, i.e. time for the healing.
5. Surgical silk loses tensile strength when exposed to moisture.
6. Monofilament sutures are preferred for vascular surgery because of minimal tissue drag and they resist harboring organisms.
7. Multifilament sutures have more tensile strength pliability, flexibility and are well suited for intestinal anastomosis.

Patient Positioning during Surgery

Proper positioning of patients during surgery is of paramount importance, and is essential in the proper exposure of the operative field. Poor positioning leads to poor access, and complications. It may also lead to pressure area damage, and nerve injuries. In this chapter, positioning of patients during common surgical procedures is described.

It is the responsibility of the surgical team to ensure that the patient's position on the table is correct. No part of the patient's body should be in contact with a metal surface if electrocautery is to be used, to avoid leaking of current from that metal contact. Excessive abduction of the upper limbs or pressure over bony prominences should be avoided to prevent neuropraxia or skin damage.

Neck Surgery

Thyroid Surgery

Patient is placed supine with the table tilted up to 15° at the head to reduce venous engorgement. A ring is placed underneath the occiput to stabilize it. The neck is extended by placing a sand bag transversely across the shoulders. Neck extension makes thyroid gland skin, platysma and strap muscles more prominent and facilitates dissection. Precautions should be taken in elderly patients and in patients with pathology of the cervical spine during extension, and hyperextension should be avoided in these cases.

Parotid Surgery

Position of the patient is supine with head resting on a ring and turned away from the side of the pathology.

Posterolateral Thoracotomy (Fig. 6.1)

Patient is turned on the unaffected side in the lateral position. The lower leg is flexed at the hip and the knee with a pillow between the legs. Table supports are used to maintain the position and additional strapping is used at the hip for stability. The upper arm is supported by a bracket in a position of 90° flexion. The lower arm is flexed and positioned underneath the head.

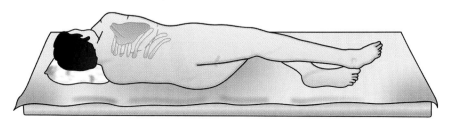

Fig. 6.1: Patient position for posterolateral thoracotomy

Lumbar Approach for Kidney (Figs 6.2 and 6.3)

Patient is turned on the unaffected side in the lateral position towards the edge of the operating table. Hip and knee next to the table are fully flexed with a pillow between the two legs. Patient is maintained in this position with a back support or by strapping. To increase the space for access, the trunk should be flexed by breaking the table, or by use of an inflatable cushion under the loin. A support for the arm prevents the shoulder from sagging forwards with consequent rotation at the waist.

Modified Radical Mastectomy

The patient lies prone with arm and forearm on the side of the surgery outstretched on an arm board to which the wrist is secured by a bandage. The forearm is supinated so that the palm faces upwards.

Anterior Resection or Abdominoperineal Resection (Fig. 6.4)

The patient is placed in the perineolithotomy position with the legs in stirrups. The patient should be brought down to the edge of the table with a sand bag under the buttocks to have proper exposure of the anal canal. The knees can be flexed but hips should be relatively extended and the thighs abducted to allow simultaneous access to both the abdomen and the perineum. A moderate degree of head down tilt (Trendelenburg) aids in dissection.

Laparotomy

Patient is placed is the supine position with arms along the side. The hands should not be placed beneath the buttocks to avoid damage to circulation and nerve supply. Be aware that the anesthetist may need access to arterial or venous

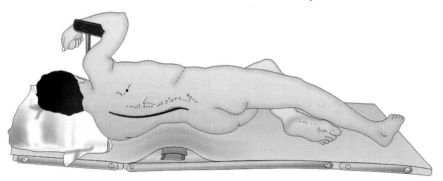

Fig. 6.2: Patient position for kidney exposure

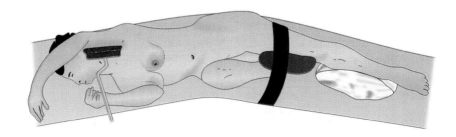

Fig. 6.3: Position of patient for kidney operations through flank approach

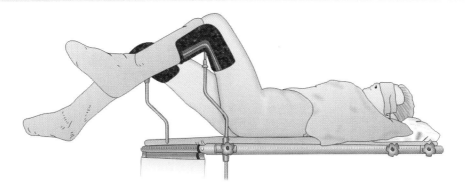

Fig. 6.4: Lloyd Davis position for abdominoperineal resection

lines during the procedure. For lower abdominal operations, the arms may be folded across the chest and secured there. The heels should be raised on a sponge rubber pad to avoid pressure on the calf muscles.

Trendelenburg's Position (Fig. 6.5)

In this position the head is tilted downwards 30°. It is frequently used in surgery of pelvis. In this position, mobile gut gravitates towards the diaphragm, so that less obstructed view of the pelvis can be obtained. Well padded shoulder rests are attached to the table in such a manner so that

pressure is exerted over the region of acromio-clavicular region to prevent the patient sliding head wards. If the pressure of shoulder head is applied on the root of the neck, brachial plexus injury may occur.

Position for Cystoscopy (Fig. 6.6)

Patient is placed with his buttocks near the end of the table with legs abducted. The thighs should be maintained at angle of 45° with the trunk. In this position the axis of the telescope is approximately horizontal when the bladder base is being examined.

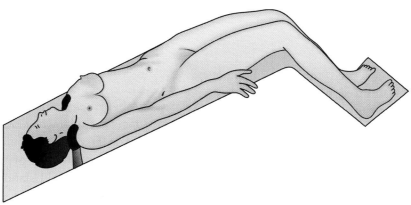

Fig. 6.5: Trendelenburg position

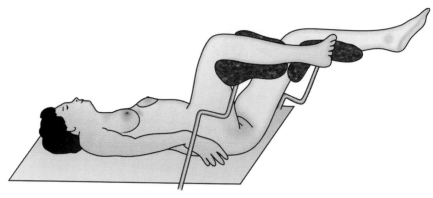

Fig. 6.6: Patient position for cystoscopy

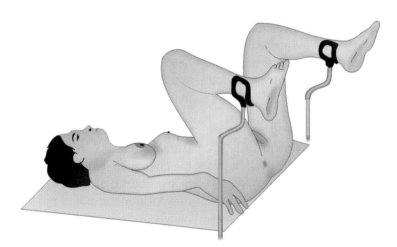

Fig. 6.7: Lithotomy position for vaginal operations

Vaginal Operations (Fig. 6.7)

Lithotomy position is used. In this position the patient's buttock are on edge of the table and rose upward with a sandbag placed across the sacrum. The knee and hip joints are flexed at 90° with legs supported on leg rest. The thighs may be slightly abducted to have space in between the thighs.

Surgeon's Position

The operating table should be of the correct height. The surgeon should work in a comfortable and relaxed posture so that he or she does not sustain back or neck muscle strain after long hours of operating. Elbows and shoulders should be kept relaxed by the proper adjustment of height of operating table as explained below. The surgeon should stand on the side which permits operating hand and arm to reach the area of pathology most easily. The surgeon should stand in a position with left foot forward and right foot back ward. In this position the surgeon's shoulder, arm and wrist are free of strain. In this position a needle is directed towards the left foot and the surgeon is able to perceive proprioceptive sensation as the needle passes through tissue and is able to feel the depth of tissue bites. Suturing in this position is known as forehand suturing and needs a strong biceps muscle for pronation and supination. Back hand motion is when an instrument is directed towards the right foot, and is required when cutting by scalpel or by electrocautery or during insertion of Lembert sutures.

Proper Height of the Operating Table

Ideal height of the operating table should be at the level of the surgeon's elbow, while operating on the abdomen or chest. If the operating table is at the level of the surgeon's elbow, the wrist is in slight dorsiflexion, which is a position of ideal function. If the height of the operating table is higher than the level of the surgeon's elbow, there will be flexion of both elbow's and wrist. In the position of wrist flexion, long extensors of the forearm and hands will be in contraction and long flexors of the forearm and hands will be in a relaxed position, but no longer in tonic balance. This imbalance increases small muscle fatigue of the hands and reduces performance of small muscles of the hand. Eye steropsis is more appropriate if the operating field is at a distance of 18 inches from the eyes.

If the operating field is a depressed body surface, within oral cavity or within pelvis, operating table should be below surgeon's elbow, so that wrist is in a position of mild ulnar deviation and relatively straight. This is a functional position of the wrist, which greatly improves dexterity and strength in the fingers.

KEY POINTS

1. Proper positioning of patient during surgery helps in the proper exposure of the operative field and facilitates in the completion of a procedure.
2. Improper position can complicate the surgery.
3. Avoid pressure on bony prominences.
4. Avoid excessive abduction of upper limb.

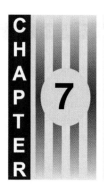

CHAPTER 7

Anastomosis in Surgery

The term anastomosis has been derived from a Greek word, with a literal meaning of 'without a mouth'. Galen (AD 131-201) used this term.

In modern day surgical practice the term anastomosis can be defined as a joining of two hollow viscera with intention to restore continuity.

The need for anastomosis arises if a portion of hollow tubular viscus has been surgically removed or destroyed by trauma, or there is a distal obstruction. In general surgery an anastomosis may involve:

1. Gut—intestinal anastomosis.
2. Vessel—vascular anastomosis.
3. Urinary tract.
4. Biliary tract or pancreatic duct.

Historical Aspects

In 1826, Antoine Lembert, a French surgeon described a seromuscular suturing technique, which has proved to be the mainstay of all gastrointestinal surgery. Nicholas Sen from USA in 1893 described a two layered technique of intestinal anastomosis, using silk and ordinary sewing needles. Halsted, a famous surgeon described a single layer closure without mucosa. Connell in 1903 from Chicago, USA described an interrupted single layer technique of gut anastomosis with knots lying intraluminally and bites going through all layers. Kocher described a two layered technique using silk and catgut. The current method of single layer extra mucosal anastomosis was advocated by Matheson of Aberdeen. Alexis Carrel in 1926 described his technique of end to end vascular anastomosis which proved to be a revolution in the field of vascular surgery.

The Ideal Anastomosis

An ideal anastomotic technique should have following features:
1. Zero leak rates.
2. Promotes early recovery of function.
3. No vascular compromise to the cut margins of a viscus.
4. Should not narrow the lumen of a viscus.
5. Easy to learn, teach and perform.
6. Technique should preferably be quick to perform.

Such an ideal technique is still to emerge.

Types of Anastomosis

1. End to end anastomosis.
2. End to side anastomosis.
3. Side to side anastomosis.

Intestinal Anastomosis

Intestinal anastomosis may involve:
1. Joining two ends of similar gut, i.e. jejuno-jejunal or ileo-ileal or colo-colic.
2. Joining two types of gut, i.e. esophagus and jejunum, stomach and jejunum, ileum and colon or rectum.

3. Joining of gut with another hollow tubular structure, e.g.
   a. Common hepatic duct and jejunun - hepaticojejunostomy.
   b. Common bile duct and duodenum - choledochoduodenostomy.
   c. Common bile duct and jejunum - choledochojejunostomy.
   d. Gallbladder and jejunum - cholecysto-jejunostomy.
   e. Pancreatic duct and jejunum - pancreatico-jejunostomy.
   f. Ureters may be implanted into an ileal conduit or in to sigmoid colon.

Vascular Anastomosis

Vascular anastomosis may involve the aorta, a peripheral artery or vein, lymphatic, coronary arteries or cerebral arteries.

Techniques of Anastomosis

Anastomosis can be:
1. Hand sewn using sutures.
2. Stapled.
3. Suture less anastomosis using laser (Nd: YAG) or tissue glue. These are still experimental. Tissue glue has been used to reinforce anastomotic suture lines.

Factors which Increase the Rate of Anastomotic Leak

Emergency surgery, if associated with hypovolemia, as in abdominal trauma with intra-abdominal bleeding. Hypovolemia compromises the splanchnic circulation, which may result in ischemia at the site of an anastomosis.

Peritonitis is a major risk factor. Most patients with peritonitis have septicemia with a systemic inflammatory response syndrome (SIRS). Here, there are high circulating levels of inflammatory

mediators, which induce excessive inflammation, (more than required for wound healing) at the site of anastomosis, rendering it friable and prone to leak.

Low hemoglobin concentration may cause decreased oxygen carrying capacity of the blood, inducing relative ischemia at the site of an anastomosis.

Malnutrition leads to low levels of serum protein and albumin, causing interstitial tissue edema, increased suture tension, and poor healing.

Previous history of irradiation. Patients who have been irradiated for malignancy have a higher incidence of anastomotic leak because irradiation induces fibrosis and a reduced blood supply.

Immunosuppressive drugs including steroids cause poor tissue healing.

Unprepared gut. An anastomosis performed on unprepared colon with a high fecal bacterial load has an increased chance of leak.

Malignancy, infection and inflammation will all impair healing.

Distal obstruction should be excluded before joining two ends. Ongoing obstruction will lead to increased tissue tension and ischemia.

Ongoing traction on an anastomosis may be seen due to mechanical tension or twists, and may also come about secondary to a narrow join, not wide enough to allow passage of fluid. This also leads to ischemia, and the possibility of anastomotic dehiscence.

The Hand Sewn Anastomosis: Technical Issues (Figs 7.1 and 7.2)

Choice of Suture Material

One should choose a suture which induces the least inflammatory reaction. The majority of sutures act as a foreign body and induce

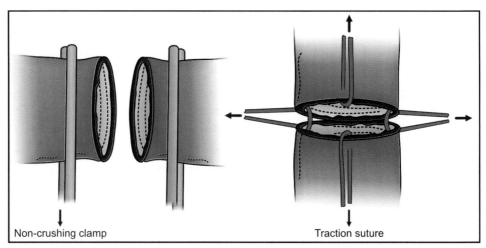

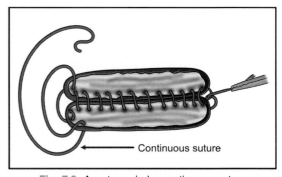

Fig. 7.1: Preparation of gut to form an anastomosis. Non-crushing clamps are applied to prevent leakage and ends are held together by traction sutures

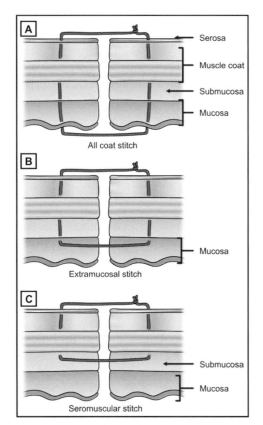

Fig. 7.2: (A) All coat stitch (above), (B) extramucosal stitch (middle) and (C) seromuscular stitch

inflammation. It has been seen that silk induces a significantly greater cellular reaction at the site an anastomosis, which persists up to 6 weeks in comparison to Polypropylene or Polyglycolic acid (Dexon) or Polyglactin. An ideal suture material for anastomosis should cause minimal inflammation and tissue reaction and should provide maximum strength during the lag phase of wound healing. Monofilaments and coated braided sutures are most effective but still not ideal.

Continuous versus Interrupted Sutures (Figs 7.3 and 7.4)

To date no randomized trial has established the superiority of one over the other but in experi-

Fig. 7.3: Anastomosis by continuous suture

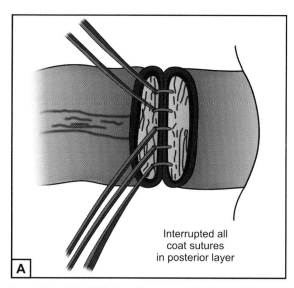

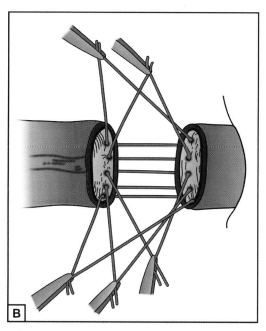

Interrupted all
coat sutures
in posterior layer

A

B

Figs. 7.4 A and B: (A) Method of anastomosis of bowel if the ends are fixed. Posterior layer stitches are applied first. (B) If one of the ends is mobile, stitches are left with ends separated until all posterior wall have been inserted. Mobile end can be railroaded along the sutures and the knots tied. This is also known as the 'telescoping' technique

mental studies using rat model, perianastomotic oxygen tension was found to be lower with continuous sutures. Narrowing of the lumen may occur with continuous sutures especially in the early phase when postoperative edema tends to tighten the suture. There may sometimes be a drawstring effect also.

Single Layer versus Double Layer Anastomosis

Double layer anastomosis which came into vogue before single layer anastomosis was traditionally thought to be more secure. However, studies have clearly shown the advantages of single layer anastomosis in the form of time saving, less narrowing of intestinal lumen, more rapid vascularization and mucosal healing, rapid increase in the strength of the anastomosis in the first few postoperative days and the early post-operative return of normal bowel function as

measured by return of bowel sounds, passage of flatus and return to oral intake.

Types of Sutured Anastomosis

There are multiple techniques in use, and the authors have described techniques which are in common use and widely accepted. One should adopt one technique and try to master it.

The Single Layer Anastomosis

There are three types:
1. A single layer interrupted extramucosal technique is preferred by many. This is mainly used for large or small bowel anastomoses.
2. Single layer interrupted full thickness. This is mainly used in biliary surgery, e.g. hepatico-jejunostomy, choledochoduodenostomy.
3. Single layer full thickness continuous technique is commonly employed for gastrojejunal

anastomosis. The continuous suture gives the advantage of hemostasis, as the gastric wall is very vascular. It also saves time.

The Two Layer Anastomosis

This consists of an inner layer taking a bite through the full thickness of the viscus. This inner layer can be continuous or interrupted depending upon the portion of viscus to be anastomosed. For small bowel, the inner layer can be continuous, but for colon the inner layer can be interrupted or continuous depending on surgeon's choice. The outer layer takes a bite through the seromuscular layer only and is usually interrupted in colonic surgery. In small bowel or stomach it is usually continuous.

The Stapled Anastomosis

Surgical stapling devices were first introduced by Hulti in 1908 but did not gain popularity because the instruments were cumbersome, unreliable and difficult to use. The past three decades have seen the development of reliable, disposable surgical stapling devices which produce consistent quality staple lines with rare technical failures. With the help of these stapling devices anastomosis at difficult sites such as low rectum, or high esophagus have become safer and more technically feasible. The drawback of stapling devices is that they are costly and the surgeon is as much reliant on technology as on his surgical skills. The main advantage of these devices is that they save time and may have a place where multiple anastomoses have to be created, e.g. in Whipple's procedure, or in radical cystectomy with ileal conduit reconstruction.

Staplers

Three types of staplers are in vogue for creating intestinal anastomosis.

1. *Transverse Anastomosis stapler (TA)*: It is the simplest type of stapler. This device places two staggered rows of B shaped staples across the bowel but does not cut them. The surgeon needs to divide the gut separately.
2. *GIA (GastroIntestinalAnastomosis) Linear Cutter*: This gastrointestinal stapler places two double staggered rows of staples and simultaneously cuts between the double rows.
3. *Circular or End to End Anastomosis stapler (EEA)*: They place a double row of staples in a circle and then cuts out the tissue within the circle of staples with a built in cylindrical knife. These staples are used for low anterior resection, gastroesophageal anastomosis or for stapled hemorrhoidopexy.

There is also an Endo GIA gun which is used for laparoscopic surgery.

Staples are made up of titanium, which causes little tissue reaction, and is non magnetic, thus enabling future MRI scanning.

Staplers can produce:
1. Functional end to end anastomosis.
2. Anatomical end to end anastomosis.
3. Side to side anastomosis.

Functional Stapled End to End Anastomosis

The steps of a functional end to end anastomosis are:
1. Place two cut ends of the bowel side to side, maintaining the orientation of mesentery.
2. Insert two limbs of GIA stapler, one each in to lumen of bowel either through an enterotomy or through the open end of the bowel. Engage the two limbs of the stapler in to each other, making sure that the mesentery of the gut does not get caught in the staple line. This can be ensured by putting a finger in between the mesenteries when the stapler is engaged.
3. The stapler is then fired to fuse the two bowel walls into a single septum and to create a

lumen between the two bowel segments by cutting between the two rows of staples.

4. Wait for one minute before removing the stapler for the hemostasis to occur (This is not always necessary but is a useful precaution).

5. Inspect the staple line for completeness and hemostasis. Under-run bleeding vessels if necessary.

A non-cutting linear stapler (TA) or a suture can be used to close the defect in gut through which GIA was inserted. Alternatively, the initial enterotomies may be placed in that part of the bowel which is to be resected.

True Anatomical End to End Anastomosis by Stapler

1. *Triangulation technique*: Cut ends of bowel are triangulated together by taking stay sutures and three linear staplers are fired in intersecting vectors to achieve complete closure. Drawback of this technique is that staple lines are everted (Fig. 7.5).

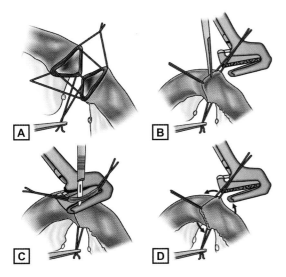

Fig. 7.5: Showing triangulation technique of end to end anastomosis by stapler:

a. Three stay sutures at three corners of divided ends of gut to triangulate the ends
b. Linear staplers applied between two stay sutures
c. Excess tissue above staple line excised
d. Gut rotated and similar process repeated between remaining stay sutures

2. Two cut ends of the bowel can be united together by using an EEA stapler, which produces a directly apposed, inverted stapled end to end anastomosis. *This is not used much now as more often end to side technique is used.*

Advantages of Stapled Anastomosis over Hand Sewn Anastomosis

1. Healing in stapled anastomosis is by primary intention but in sutured anastomosis it is by secondary intention.

2. Titanium staples used in anastomosis provoke minimal inflammatory response.

3. They provide support to the cut surfaces in lag phase (weakest phase of healing).

4. Stapling may shorten operating time especially in low pelvic anastomosis, or in the thorax, or high abdomen.

5. After a cancer resection, recurrence at the staple line is much less than at suture line because suture materials produce a more pronounced cellular proliferation than staples.

Inverted Suture Line versus Everted Suture Line

An inverted suture line is found to be better than an everted suture line in terms of bursting pressure, rate of healing and degree of inflammation. An inverted suture line has a greater aesthetic appeal although this has little relevance to healing.

Testing Anastomoses

In certain situations where an anastomosis is performed in a difficult situation, e.g. low anorectal anastomosis, esophagogastric anastomosis or where the anastomosis is complex as in the creation of an ileoanal pouch, testing of anastomoses is important. Anastomoses can be tested by following methods:

The Underwater Test

This performed in cases of low anterior resection (LAR) or in cases of esophagogastric anastomosis.

A soft non crushing clamp is applied on gastric side or on sigmoid colon just distal to the anastomoses. Pelvic cavity or left subdiaphragmatic space is filled with saline. Air is insufflated from anal opening in case of LAR or nasogastric tube in case of esophagogastric anastomoses. If there is no bubbling of air into the saline the anastomoses is airtight, and presumed to be safe.

The Methylene Blue Test

This test is performed in cases of gastric pouch surgery for obesity. After completion of the anastomoses, methylene blue is injected through a nasogastric tube . There should not be any leak of methylene blue from the gastrojejunostomy.

Protecting an Anastomosis

Nasogastric Decompression

Routine nasogastric decompression is not mandatory after lower intestinal anastomosis unless there is a significant paralytic ileus with abdominal distension, or there is gastric dilatation or the patient is vomiting.

In upper gastrointestinal anastomoses, e.g. gastrojejunostomy or gastroduodenal anastomosis nasogastric suction is essential for 3-5 days to avoid any tension on the suture line caused by retention of gastric secretions. Gastric motility takes around 72 hours to recover and a nasogastric tube may prevent acute gastric dilatation.

Stents are left across anastomoses following hepaticojejunostomy and pancreaticojejunostomy to prevent bile or pancreatic leaks.

A nasogastric tube is left after every emergency laparotomy.

An unwanted side effect of nasogastric tube placement is discomfort in the pharynx, and difficulty coughing.

Abdominal Drains after Intestinal Anastomosis

The ability of abdominal drainage to "protect" an anastomosis has been challenged by Yates. The peritoneal cavity cannot be drained effectively by a single drain due to the rapid development of adhesions and sealing of the drainage tract. Severe inflammatory reactions have been shown to occur around drains.

An intra-abdominal drain after anterior resection or ileo-anal anastomosis is kept in the pelvis because there is higher than usual incidence of fluid collections in the pelvis after these operations.

General Principles of Intestinal Anastomosis

1. There should not be any disparity between the two ends of lumen to be joined together. If one end is narrower than other, it can be enlarged by giving a back cut around antimesenteric border sometimes also known as "fish mouthing" of the end.
2. To prevent leakage of contents and to steady the two ends, either non crushing clamps can be applied across the gut or stay sutures can be taken at the end.
3. Three types of suture can be used for uniting gut:
   a. All coat stitches in which bites are taken through all layers of gut. This was advocated by William Halsted (1852-1922) (Fig. 7.2).
   b. In extra mucosal or sero-submucosal technique all layers are included except mucosa. Submucosa is the strongest layer, as it contains plenty of collagen tissue (Fig. 7.2).
   c. In seromuscular stitch bites are taken through serosa and part of the muscular

layer. This was described by a surgeon from Paris (Antoine Lembert). This stitch is also known as a Lembert stich. It is generally used in a second layer to strengthen the first layer.

Basic Arterial Surgical Techniques

Arterial surgery is generally undertaken to:
1. Repair arteries
2. Reconstruct arteries.

Arterial surgery like all other anastomoses should be undertaken in optimum conditions with good light, good exposure and good control of bleeding.

Precautions during Arterial Anastomosis

1. Handle arteries gently, and veins with extreme gentleness.
2. Vessels should be held by the periarterial or adventitial tissue whenever possible to avoid trauma to the vessel wall.
3. If one needs to handle the arterial wall directly, use the tip of closed dissecting forceps.
4. Use a suture which passes easily without causing trauma and which causes least tissue reaction. A monofilament suture such as Prolene is an excellent choice.
5. Round bodied needles are used for the majority of vessels but taper cut needles are better for dense graft material or for heavily diseased arteries.
6. The needle should be passed from inside to out - from intima to adventitia. This pins down atherosclerotic plaques to prevent the formation of intimal flaps which may lead to dissection, embolization or thrombosis.
7. Suture material should not be held with dissecting forceps, needle holders or forceps, all of which can damage the thread.
8. Knots should be hand tied.
9. When a needle has to be passed from adventitia to intima (from outside to inside)

the intima should be supported against the vessel wall as the needle is inserted.
10. The needle should pass at right angles to the arterial wall and should be passed through the wall along the arc of the needle *without deploying excessive force*, to avoid splitting or tearing the delicate vessel wall.
11. The suture line should be smooth and everted. This provides good intimal apposition and prevents platelet aggregation on the suture line.
12. When suturing a transverse defect in an artery, start from the outside in on the upstream side and from inside out on the downstream side, in order to avoid dissection of intima from the arterial wall by turbulent blood flow. This may produce a dissecting aneurysm especially in aorta.
13. Vascular sutures may be:
    a. *Unlocked continuous*: Continuous unlocked sutures form a spiral around the artery, which tightens with each distending pulsation of the vessel. A tightened spiral reduces the likelihood of leakage. If a continuous suture is locked, the spiral effect will be lost and the suture will not become tightened with arterial pulsations.
    b. *Interrupted sutures*: These are used for small vessels to reduce the risk of stenosis. They are used in children, to permit the growth of vessel circumference along with the growth of child. A draw back of interrupted sutures is increased risk of bleeding when the sutures separate with distension of vessels.
    c. *Mattress sutures*: Mattress sutures are not generally used in vascular surgery because they tend to narrow the lumen. Sometimes a single mattress suture may be used to initiate eversion or in case of diseased arteries when there is danger of simple sutures cutting out.

The Arteriotomy (Fig. 7.6)

An arteriotomy should be longitudinal to permit visualization of the vessel lumen and to permit approaches to branches of the artery. In cases of vessels less than 4 mm in diameter, where an arteriotomy has been made only for embolectomy, a transverse incision can be made which has the advantage of less narrowing of the lumen. Closure of an arteriotomy is performed by continuous unlocking suture with intimal apposition and eversion of cut edges. The non-intimal layer of the arterial wall should not come in contact with flowing blood unless an endarterectomy has been performed. As it may be difficult to include all layers in the suture at the end of the arteriotomy, two appropriately sized double ended arterial sutures are used. Closure is started from either end with both needles passing from inside out. Sutures are tied and secure in a rubber shod forcep. Suturing is continued from both ends using fine, evenly spaced stitches, until one reaches the apex of the vessel. The two sutures from both ends are then tied at the apex.

Vein Patch Graft

Vein patch grafts are used to close an arteriotomy if it is likely that simple closure will result in narrowing of the lumen of the artery. The chances of narrowing after simple closure of an arteriotomy are greater if the artery is smaller than the diameter

of the common femoral artery or if the closure of a diseased segment of artery is performed.

Vein patches are usually from autologous long saphenous vein taken from the ankle or from one of the groin tributaries. Proximal long saphenous vein should not be sacrificed as it may be utilized for future vascular reconstructive procedures. If suitable vein is not available then a patch of Dacron or expanded polytetrafluoroethylene (e-PTFE) can be used.

Steps of Arteriotomy Closure Using Vein Patch Graft (Fig. 7.7)

1. Prepare a suitable vein patch graft or synthetic graft patch by trimming one end to form a

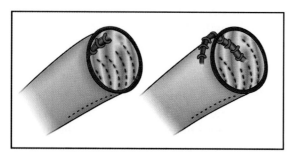

Fig. 7.6: Arteriotomy in a small size vessel should be longitudinal, because clot if formed on suture line will cause less narrowing of lumen if formed around longitudinal suture line in comparison to a transverse suture line

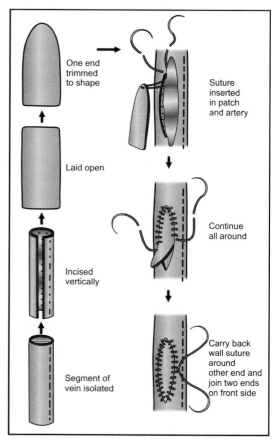

One end trimmed to shape

Suture inserted in patch and artery

Laid open

Continue all around

Incised vertically

Segment of vein isolated

Carry back wall suture around other end and join two ends on front side

Fig. 7.7: Steps of vein patch insertion to close an arteriotomy

round ellipse that will fit into the end of the incision. Do not cut the other end, because the excess portion can be used to handle the patch without damaging the intima.

2. Take a suitable size double needled Prolene suture on a round bodied needle. Insert both needles from outside in the sides of the vein patch. Pass needles from inside to outside through the one cut end of the incision, in such a manner so that suture is halved. Tie the suture.

3. Continue taking continuous over and over sutures on the back the wall and front wall using one needle each.

4. Once the half way point is reached, trim the end of the vein patch to a rounded ellipse to fit the remaining defect. While trimming the other end of vein patch, make sure that tension on suture is not loosened.

5. After trimming the vein patch, continue suturing on both sites until you meet at the apex of the defect where both sutures should emerge on the outer surface of the artery to be tied.

End to End Anastomosis (Figs 7.8 and 7.9)

General Principles

1. Bevel the ends of the arteries to be united to avoid narrowing except in large vessels. Bevelling can be done by cutting the ends obliquely.

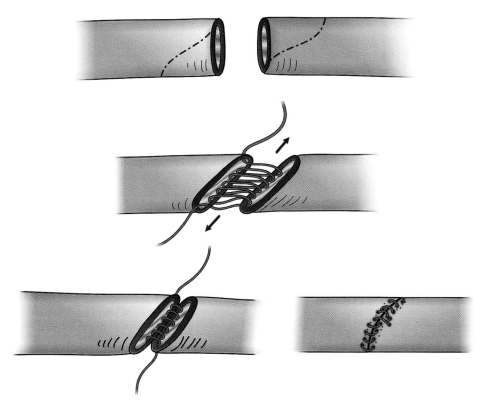

Fig. 7.8: Method of performing end to end arterial anastomosis.
Ends are bevelled by cutting obliquely before performing anastomosis to prevent narrowing

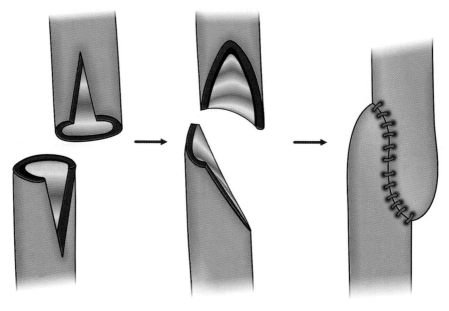

Fig. 7.9: End to end arterial anastomosis. Ends are bevelled to avoid narrowing

2. Use continuous unlocked sutures except in children to avoid hampering of growth or in very small or delicate vessels.
3. Pediatric vessels are more prone to go in to spasm, so handle them gently.
4. Place sutures from outside to inside on the upstream side and from inside to outside on down stream side. There are two techniques of performing vascular anastomosis.

a. *Anchoring suture technique*: First anchoring sutures are placed and the vessel is rotated, so that all sutures are placed from outside.
b. *Parachuting technique*.

Anchoring Suture Technique (Fig. 7.10)

Three anchoring sutures are placed at equal distance around the whole circumference of the vessels. These sutures are used for rotating the vessel for the purpose of gaining access. This technique is very good where mobility of vessels is not restricted.

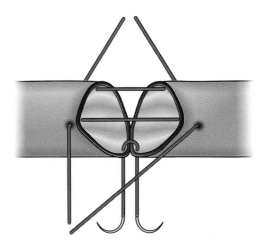

Fig. 7.10: Anchoring suture technique for vascular anastomosis

Parachuting Technique (Fig. 7.11)

This is useful if the mobility of vessels is restricted by branches. In this technique the vessels are kept apart. A posterior row of continuous unlocked

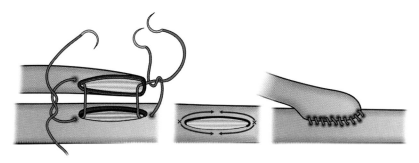

Fig. 7.11: Parachuting technique

sutures is applied first using a double needled suture starting from the posterior midline and working outwards alternatively on each side, continuing around to the front. Ends of the vessels are then gently drawn or parachuted together. Parachuting is only possible if a frictionless polypropylene suture is used.

KEY POINTS

1. The ideal anastomotic technique is still to emerge.
2. Every surgical trainee must learn and master hand sewn anastomotic techniques.
3. A stapled anastomosis is not superior to a hand sewn one, but it may save time.
4. Staplers add to the cost of surgery.
5. There is no difference in leak rate between continuous and interrupted sutures following intestinal anastomosis.
6. Vascularity of resected ends of gut should be ensured before joining them.
7. Abdominal drainage after intestinal anastomosis should be avoided except in cases of peritonitis or trauma.
8. Single layer anastomosis scores over double layer technique in terms of time saving, less luminal narrowing and early return of postoperative bowel function.
9. During arterial anastomosis, hold arteries by periarterial or advential tissue to avoid trauma to arterial wall.
10. Monofilament suture, i.e. prolene with round body needle is the suture of choice for arterial anastomosis.
11. For an arterial anastomosis the needle should pass from inside to outside to prevent formation of intimal flaps and to fix any atherosclerotic plaque.

Instrument Handling

INTRODUCTION

Every surgeon must be aware of the proper functioning of common instruments used in day to day surgical practice. It is very important to learn the proper way of handling instruments, so that injury to the surgical team or patient can be avoided, and malfunctioning of instruments can be prevented.

In this chapter instrument handling techniques are described.

Broad Classification of Instruments

Instruments for Cutting

1. Scissors
2. Scalpel

Instruments for Grasping

1. Thumb forceps (toothed/non-toothed)
2. Artery forceps
3. Babcock forceps
4. Ellis forceps

Instrument for Suturing

1. Needle holders

The Scalpel

This is the most basic surgical instrument. It comprises of a handle and blade. Blades are disposable and handles reusable.

The handle is commonly known as a BP handle after Bard Parker, the inventor. It comes in two sizes 3, and 4. The number 3 handle will accommodate a small sized surgical blade of numbers 10 to 15. The number 4 handle will accommodate larger blades ranging from size 18 to 24.

Handling

A surgical knife or scalpel should be transferred from scrub nurse to surgeon and *vice versa* in a kidney tray, not from hand to hand, in order to avoid injuries from the very sharp blade (Figs 8.1 and 8.2).

Never try to load or unload the blade on to the handle by hand. This should only be attempted with the blade being held in forceps.

To load the blade onto a scalpel handle, hold the blade in artery forceps near the base of cutting edge and advance it in to the scalpel, until the lower end of the blade fits into a groove on the handle and you hear a click (Fig. 8.3).

To unload the blade, hold the base of the blade and then lift it up and pull it out of the groove, again using forceps (Fig. 8.4).

The scalpel can be held as a table knife for a skin incision. The knife is held at 30 degrees or less from the horizontal in a pronated hand, between thumb and middle finger with index finger at base of the blade on the upper surface to apply and control pressure. Grip is strengthened

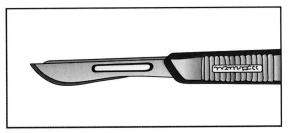

Fig. 8.1: Number 10 surgical blade

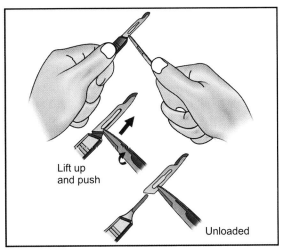

Fig. 8.4: Steps for unloading a blade
from a scalpel handle

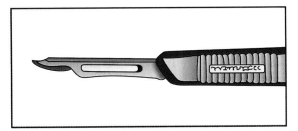

Fig. 8.2: Number 15 surgical blade

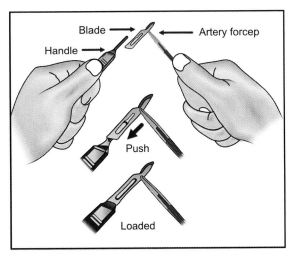

Fig. 8.3: Steps for loading a blade on scalpel handle

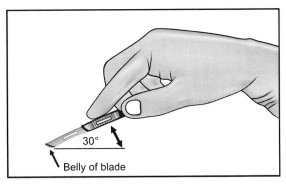

Fig. 8.5: Method of holding scalpel with no. 10 blade

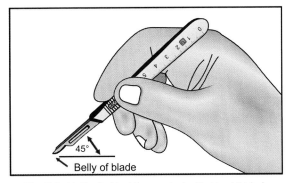

Fig. 8.6: Method of holding scalpel with No. 15 blade

by wrapping the ring and little finger around the handle, which rests on the hypothenar muscles (Fig. 8.5).

For a small, precise cut, the scalpel is held like a pen (Fig. 8.6).

It is a good surgical practice to mark the incision with skin marking pencil or with the back of the blade before actually incising it.

Blade numbers 20 to 24 have a wider shaft and are used for larger incisions and dissection. Number 15 blades have a narrower shaft and are used for smaller incisions, for example when making port sites for laparoscopic surgery, or when removing small skin lesions.

The number 11 blade is also known as a stab knife, and is used for incision and drainage of abscesses and to incise skin for inserting drains.

The Scissors

Scissors are very useful and versatile instruments. They can be used for:
1. Tissue dissection.
2. Undermining skin or raising skin flaps.
3. Dividing tissue.
4. Cutting sutures.
5. Cutting gauze, meshes or other surgical materials.
6. Opening tissue planes.
7. Assisting the surgeon in the palpation of tissues.
8. Probing cavities

Types of Scissor

1. Dissecting scissors with a blunt tip.
2. Cutting scissors with a sharp tip.

Scissors have two blades—one is moving and cutting, while the other is stationary. Scissors can be straight or curved. Cutting scissors are known as Mayo's scissors and are used for cutting heavy fascia and sutures. Lighter dissecting scissors such as Metzenbaum or McIndoe's scissors are used for dissection and cutting delicate tissue. They have a longer handle to blade ratio.

Handling (Fig. 8.7)

Each blade has a ring at the end, also known as a bow. For holding scissors, the hand should be in

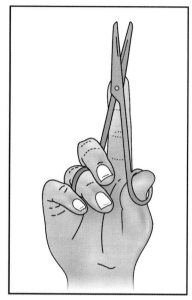

Fig. 8.7: Method of holding scissor

a mid pronated position. The distal phalanx of the thumb should go into the ring of the moving blade and the distal phalanx of the ring finger into the other ring. The ring should never go beyond the distal interphalangeal joint. The tip of the index finger should rest over the joint of the blades and middle finger should wrap around the handle to steady it. While dividing tissues or sutures in a cavity, the scissor blades should rest over the index finger of the non-dominant hand to steady them, and to minimize tremors.

In a vertical direction scissors cut from near to far and in a transverse direction from dominant to the non-dominant side. If you want to cut from non-dominant to dominant side or from far to near, it is advisable to use a scalpel unless skilled in using scissors in either hand. Some surgeons point the direction of blades towards the elbow while cutting from left to right with the right hand.

Tissue Holding Forceps or Thumb Forceps (Fig. 8.8)

These consist of two shafts held together at one end with a spring device that holds the shafts

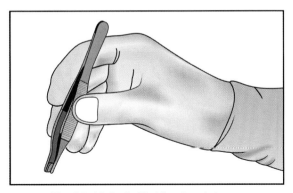

Fig. 8.8: Method of holding thumb forcep

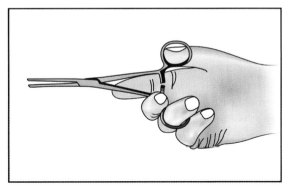

Fig. 8.9: Method of holding artery forcep

open. The tips of forceps can be smooth, serrated or have teeth.

For holding skin, tough fascia or tendon, thumb forceps with a toothed tip are used.

For holding delicate structures, thumb forceps with smooth tips or serrated tips are used.

The main use of forceps is to retract, stabilize or grasp tissue. Forceps are held like a pen between thumb and middle finger in the non dominant hand with index finger to stabilize the forceps. Non toothed thumb forceps with round tips may be used for dissection. The closed forceps tips are inserted into the desired plane and when the blades spring open, the tissue plane also opens.

Artery Forceps (Hemostatic Forceps, Hemostats) (Figs 8.9 and 8.10)

These were devised by the celebrated French Surgeon, Ambroise Paré (1510-1590). His design was modified and improved by the introduction of a locking mechanism by Thomas Spencer Wells (1818-1897).

Artery forceps are mainly used for holding bleeding vessels before they are occluded by a ligature or cauterized. They can also be used for dissection or for holding tough structures, such as fascia. They are pointed at one end, with rings at the ends of two shafts, linked with a hinge in the middle, and a ratchet to lock the blades.

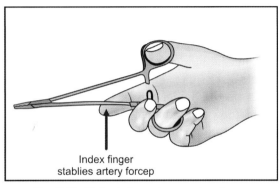

Index finger
stablies artery forcep

Fig. 8.10: Method of opening an artery forcep

Handling

The instrument is held like a needle holder. For locking the ratchet, handles are compressed. For unlocking, first lightly compress, and then separate the handles at a right angle to the hinge action. One should be able to lock and unlock them with either hand. For holding blood vessels, curved forceps are used with the concavity upwards and the tips extending beyond the vessel.

For ligating blood vessels which have been held by artery forceps, the assistant holds the forcep tips up and visible, so that surgeon can pass a ligature around the vessel. When the first half of the knot is being tied, the assistant gently releases and removes the artery forceps, at the surgeon's verbal request, and not before.

Artery forceps are available in different shapes and sizes. They can be curved or straight. Small sized artery forceps with fine tips are also known as Mosquito forceps. Other types include Kelly's, Spencer Well's or Roberts. The Spencer Wells hemostatic forceps blades are usually half of the length of the shaft and have transverse serrations along the whole length of the blade with conical tips. In Kelly's clamps, the blades are short and transverse serrations are present along the whole length.

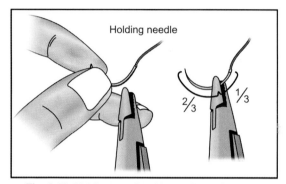

Fig. 8.11: Holding needle with needle holder at the junction of 2/3 and 1/3rd from it's tip

Needle Holders (Figs 8.11 to 8.13)

These are used for holding and driving needles through tissue. It may also be called a needle driver. The needle holder is held in the same way as surgical scissors.

A needle holder can be differentiated from artery forceps by smaller, short blunt blades, cris cross serrations and a groove in the center of the blade. A Mayo needle holder with a ratchet similar in design to that of artery forceps is commonly used.

Plastic surgeons may use a smaller needle holder without a locking device and with a scissor at the tip. This type of needle holder was devised by Sir Harold Gilles, the famous British plastic surgeon.

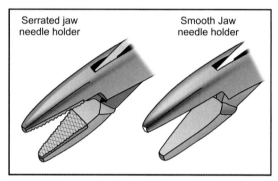

Fig. 8.12: Serrated jaw and smooth jaw needle holder

Handling

Needle holders grip needles with especially designed jaws. Needles should be held 1/3rd of the way along the needle shaft from the suture material. Pronation and supination (backhand and forehand) are used to drive the needle into tissue. During pronation/supination movement, the needle holder rotates in its long axis and moves the needle in a curved plane through tissue. A curved needle must be driven along its own curved shape through tissue, and will bend if gripped incorrectly, or driven in the wrong plane.

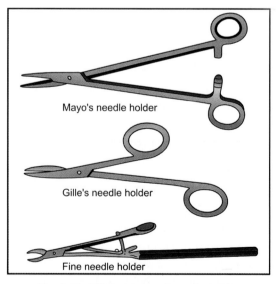

Fig. 8.13: Different types of needle holders

Needles should be gripped at the tip of a needle holder, with a 90 to 105° angle with the shaft of the needle holder. The needlepoint should face the non-dominant hand and point upwards.

When suturing in a deep cavity such as the pelvis, it is a good practice to use long needle holders in order to avoid hands blocking vision of the needle and tissues

Whilst tying knots by hand, a needle holder with needle (mounted needle holder) may be kept on one side, in order to avoid needle prick. Some surgeons palm the needle holder between first interspaces between thumb and second metacarpal, but this requires practice.

If it is essential to change the direction of a needle while stitching from right to left and *vice versa*, instead of taking out the needle from needle holder, turn the needle up side down inside needle holder and then rotate the needle holder through 180° (Fig. 8.15).

Retractors (Figs 8.14 to 8.17)

Retractors are instruments used to pull tissue aside to display a surgical field. They are especially useful when working in a close cavity such as the pelvis or on a deeply placed organ such as kidney or oesophagus. Retractors are available in various sizes and shapes. Some are self retaining and others are hand held.

The basic principal of retraction is that tissues should be displaced laterally out of the operative field. One should safeguard the underlying structure to be retracted against injury by putting sponge or gauze beneath the retractor. An assistant who is retracting should be allowed to relax between surgical manoeuvres in order to avoid tiring and cramp. Retractors are used for traction, counter traction or for both.

Traction is defined as pulling the tissue in one direction. Counter traction may be applied with

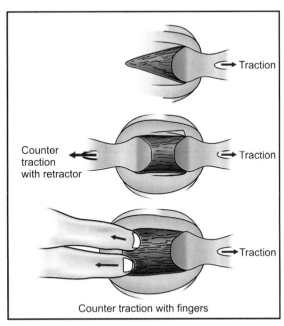

Fig. 8.14: Traction by retractor and counter traction either by retractor or by fingers

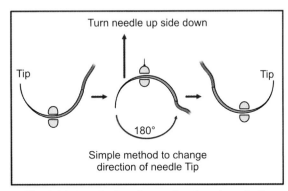

Fig. 8.15: A method to change direction of needle tip

another retractor or by hand, for example using a Deaver's retractor to retract the liver, and hand to retract the duodenum and bile duct in displaying the cystic duct structures.

Retractors can be:
– Superficial retractors
– Deep retractors
– Self retaining retractors

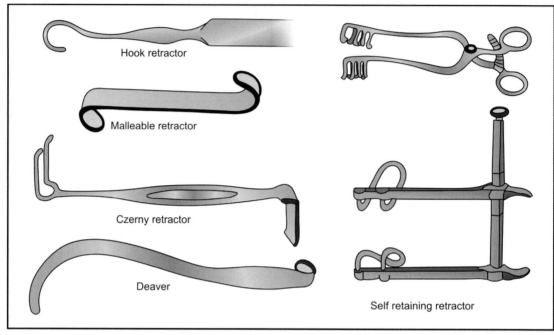

Fig. 8.16: Different types of retractors

Superficial Retractors

1. *Langenbeck's retractor*: It has a long handle and small solid blade. It is commonly used for hernia surgery or in any superficial surgery to retract fascia or aponeurosis.
2. *Czerny's retractor*: It has thick small blade on one side and biflanged hook on other side in opposite direction. It is used during abdominal closure, during appedicectomy.

Deep Retractors

1. *Morris retractor*: It is used for abdominal wall retraction.
2. *Deaver's retractor*: It is used to retract liver, spleen and other abdominal organs. It is an atraumatic and has broad gently curved blade.
3. *Doyen's retractor*: It is used during pelvic operations.

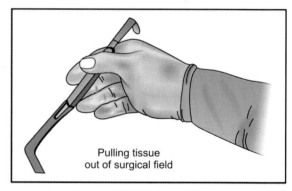

Fig. 8.17: Langenback's retractor

Principals of Retraction

1. Retraction should be gentle.
2. Injury to underlying structures should be avoided during retraction.
3. During retraction of the abdominal wall, retraction should be upwards.

Clamps (Fig. 8.18)

Beside artery forceps, used to permanently seal vessels, there are many other clamps with different uses in surgery.

Vascular clamps—for example Bulldog clamp, Pot's arterial clamp and Satinsky clamps. These are designed to occlude vessels temporarily without damaging them.

Intestinal clamps—which can be crushing or non-crushing. Crushing clamps are used during intestinal resection to control bleeding and leakage from the divided bowel and to create a clean edge for anastomosis. They may be used to hold the divided ends of gut whilst suturing.

Non-crushing intestinal clamps may be used to display a viscus, and to prevent intestinal spillage. They are not totally atraumatic, and should be applied and locked up to one ratchet only.

Tissue Holding Forceps (Fig. 8.19)

Beside thumb forceps, there are other tissue holding forceps, e.g. Babcock forceps, Allis forceps and Lane's tissue forceps. Babcock forceps are non-traumatic and are used for holding gut, ureter or bladder. Allis forceps have long blades with gaps between the blades. There are sharp teeth at the tip of the blades with grooves in between. When these forceps are locked, the tooth of one blade fits into the groove of the other blade and *vice versa*. These are used for holding tough structures such as skin, deep fascia or aponeurosis.

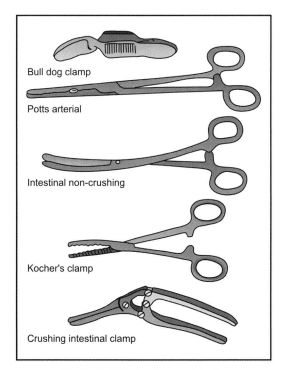

Fig. 8.18: Different types of clamps

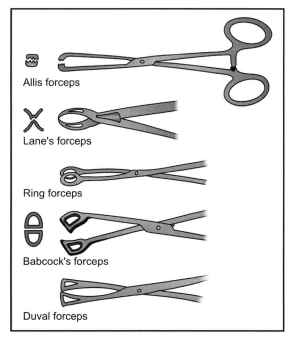

Fig. 8.19: Different types of tissue holding forceps

Lane's tissue forceps are heavy and traumatising, with curved fenestrated blades. At the tip, there is a heavy tooth in one blade with a groove in the other blade. In the closed position, the tooth fits into the groove. This may be used for grasping a fibrous salivary gland during excision or breast tissue during mastectomy. They may also be used to grip the spermatic cord during hernia repair, and may still occasionally be used to replace a lost towel clip.

KEY POINTS

1. Proper handling of instruments is of paramount importance for optimum surgical outcome.
2. Hold a scalpel like a pen if a small precise incision is planned.
3. If a long incision on skin is planned, a scalpel may be held like a table knife.
4. No 3 BP handle accommodates size 10 to 15 surgical blades.
5. No 4 BP handle accommodates size 18 to 24 surgical blades.
6. Scissors can be used for a variety of functions ranging from tissue dissection, raising skin flaps and opening tissue planes.
7. Hold scissors in a mid pronated hand position with distal phalanx of thumb into the ring of the moving blade and distal phalanx of ring finger into the other ring. Ring should never go beyond distal interphalangeal joint.
8. In a needle holder, the needle should be held at the junction of 2/3 and 1//3 from the tip of needle.
9. Needles should never be pushed through tissue, rather use the movement of supination and pronation of the hand to drive the needle through tissue along its own shape.

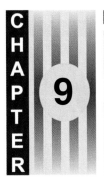

Drains in Surgery

9

DEFINITION

A drain is a device to prevent collection of fluid in a cavity or a closed space. This space may be anatomical or created by surgical dissection. The fluid may be pus, blood, serum, urine, biliary or pancreatic secretions, intestinal contents, chyle or air.

The following are indications for inserting drains—the list is not exhaustive, and some indications are relative.

Drainage of Pus

a. After incision and drainage of any large abscess, e.g. subdiaphragmatic
b. Drainage of empyema of thorax
c. Drainage of empyema of gallbladder
d. After pancreatic necrosectomy or drainage of infected pseudocyst.
e. After surgery for peritonitis (Controversial).

Drainage of Blood

a. Hemothorax
b. After laparotomy for hemoperitoneum secondary to any etiology
c. Drainage of scrotum after operation for large hydrocele or hernia.
d. Drainage of subcutaneous space following mastectomy, thyroid surgery or open surgery for large incisional hernias.
e. After liver surgery including cholecystectomy.
f. Radical excision of pelvic tumors

Drainage of Intestinal Contents/Bile

a. After anastomosis of intestinal viscus where there is increased risk of leak, e.g. in the malnourished or septic patient, or where blood supply is threatened. A drain may herald a leak, leading to early re-laparotomy, or may be its primary management.
b. After common bile duct injuries during cholecystectomy.
c. After restorative surgery for bile duct strictures.

Drainage of Pancreatic Juice

1. After pancreatic resection
2. After pancreatic trauma.

Drainage of Chyle

1. Chylothorax
2. Chylocele.

Drainage of Urine

Surgery on the urinary tract where urinary leak is likely to occur.

Drainage of Air

Pneumothorax

Indications for drainage can be classified as follows:

Emergency

- Tension pneumothorax
- Pericardial tamponade

- Solid organ abscess
- Intraperitoneal abscess
- Skin or subcutaneous abscess.

Therapeutic

- Hemothorax
- Empyema
- Pseudocyst.

Prophylactic (Relative Indications only)

- Post-thoracic surgery – cardiopulmonary or esophageal.
- Post-abdominal surgery (including urological procedures).
- Post-orthopedic joint surgery.
- Head and neck surgery.

   Any operation involving extensive skin or muscle flaps, e.g. mastectomy, incisional hernia, latissimus dorsi flap.

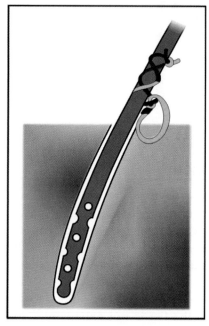

Fig. 9.1: Tube drain with multiple side holes

Types of Drains

Tube Drains (Fig. 9.1)

Tube drains permit the formation of a closed drainage system, as they can be connected to bags or reservoirs. There are multiple holes at the end of the drain. Suction can be applied at the end of the tube drains.

Sheet Drains (Figs 9.2 and 9.3)

These consist if corrugated silicone material, or of sheets forming parallel tubes (Yeates drain), in which fluid passes through and around the tubes. These drains are either exteriorized through a main wound or via a separate stab wound. They are fixed by either suture to the skin or passing a large safety pin through drain and skin. Neither is commonly used now.

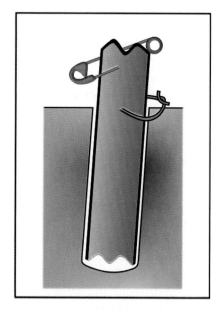

Fig. 9.2: Corrugated sheet drain

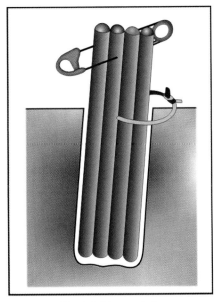

Fig. 9.3: Yeates drain

Gauze Packs and Ribbon Gauze Wicks (Fig. 9.4)

Gauze packs are sheets of sterile cotton gauze placed on a raw surface where discharge is expected to occur over a wide area, e.g. in an abscess cavity or after laying open of a fistulous tract. Gauze acts by capillary action, soaking up secretions. Packs may be soaked in saline with a lubricant such as liquid paraffin. Antiseptic agents such as Betadine may also be used.

Dry gauze packs are more effective but tend to adhere to raw areas and are difficult to remove. This may lead to pain and bleeding.

If a cavity is deep and discharge cannot be brought to the surface, it can be drained by a wick of folded gauze which is passed down. To be fully effective, it should be moist. Sometimes wicks can be passed through a thin walled latex tube, known as 'cigarette drain'. The latex tube prevents the wick becoming adherent to tissues (Fig. 9.5).

Drain can be made of:
1. *Latex rubber*: It is soft but excites a profound inflammatory reaction within 24 hours and renders them totally ineffective.
2. *PVC*: It is much less reactive and more efficient. They are firm and more unyielding but tend to harden with prolonged use especially when come in contact with bile.

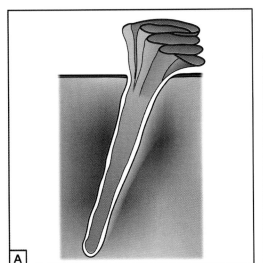
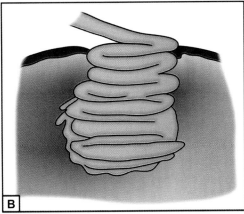

Figs 9.4A and B: Wound being packed by a folded gauze piece (A) or a ribbon pack. (B) This is usually performed to drain a cavity

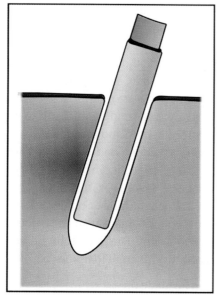

Fig. 9.5: 'Cigarette' drain. This is formed by passing a folded gauze piece or a ribbon pack through a finger glove stalk or a thin walled rubber tube

3. *Silicon*: It is the best material for drains because it is least reactive, more pliable and do not get hardened with prolonged use.

Types of Drainage System

1. *Open drainage*: In this system Penrose drain, multitubular drain or corrugated drain is used. The drain is taken out through the main operative wound or via a separate stab wound stitched to the skin or secured by a safety pin. This is then covered by a surgical dressing pad. This type of drain increases the incidence of wound infection and disseminates infection to other patients in surgical ward.

2. *Closed siphon drainage*: In this system a tube drain is connected to a drainage bag. The drainage bag has a one way valve at the entrance and a drainage tap at the opposite end. The tap allows daily emptying without disconnection.

3. *Closed suction drainage*: In this system firm polyethylene tubes are connected to portable suction devices. Some devices utilise low pressure vacuum (-100 to -150 mm Hg), i.e. Romovac or Reliavac. Others utilize high pressure negative suction (-300 to 500 mm Hg), i.e. Redivac. They are particularly used for drainage of dissected spaces, e.g. after incisional hernia repair. They should not be used inside the peritoneal cavity as they can cause injury to gut due to negative suction.

4. *Sump suction drainage*: These drainage systems also employ negative suction but they have parallel air vent which prevent adjacent soft tissue being sucked in to the lumen. They are made of either silicon or PVC. They are useful in management of small bowel fistula or pancreatic fistula.

KEY POINTS

1. A drain is a device to prevent collection of undesired or unwanted fluid in a cavity or a closed space.
2. It can be used to drain pus, blood, intestinal contents, chyle or air.
3. Absolute indications for placing drains are tension pneumothorax, hemothorax, after pancreatic necrosectomy and in a localized collection of pus.
4. Drain may be harmful after appendicectomy.
5. A drain itself can cause complications by erosion into viscera.
6. Drains often reassure the surgeon rather than draining anything.
7. Whenever in doubt about hemostasis always put a drain.

Minimal Access Surgery

DEFINITION

Minimal access surgery can be defined as the application of modern technology to minimize the trauma of surgical access, without compromising the exposure of the surgical site, or the safety of the patient.

INTRODUCTION

Wickman and Fitzpatrick in 1990 coined the term "minimally invasive surgery" in order to promote techniques with reduced operative trauma. Cuschieri in 1992 coined the term **minimal access surgery (MAS)**, which in many regards is more accurate and descriptive.

The following techniques are included under the umbrella of MAS:
1. Laparoscopic surgery
2. Thoracoscopy
3. Endoluminal endoscopy
4. Perivisceral endoscopy
5. Arthroscopy
6. Combined approach.

In this chapter the basics of laparoscopic surgery only will be discussed.

The Advantages of Laparoscopic Surgery

In laparoscopy, retraction is provided by a low pressure CO_2 pneumoperitoneum (8-15 mm Hg), which is gently and evenly applied to the abdominal musculature and diaphragm, in contrast to the localized pressure of a mechanical retractor. Incisions are very small at 5-10 mm, and therefore less painful.

The incidence of hypothermia and evaporative fluid loss during laparoscopic surgery is much less because there is no exposure of the abdominal contents to the atmosphere.

There is a lower incidence of postoperative intestinal adhesions after laparoscopy due to minimal handling of gut. This leads to less serosal tears, less adhesions, and a reduced incidence of postoperative paralytic ileus.

In the past there was a saying that "big surgeons make big incisions". A large incision may, however, be the cause of morbidity, increasing the likelihood of:

Pain (Acute and Chronic)

- Infection
- Bleeding
- Incisional hernia.

Any of the above may prevent early ambulation and recovery. Delay in mobility may lead to deep vein thrombosis, pulmonary embolism, or pulmonary consolidation.

Causes of Pain in Open Surgery

1. Trauma of cutting muscles and other structures such as nerve, aponeurosis or fascia.
2. Mechanical retractors leading to localized bruising or ischemia to muscle or nerve caused by sustained pressure.

A large incision is more painful than a small one.

Contraindications to Laparoscopic Surgery

1. Unwilling patient
2. Untrained surgeon
3. Untreated bleeding disorders
4. Patient in shock.

Relative Contraindications to Laparoscopic Surgery

1. History of previous extensive abdominal surgery
2. Known intra-abdominal adhesions
3. Bowel obstruction, organomegaly
4. Pregnancy.

New Skills to be Learned by the Laparoscopic Surgeon

Mechanical Limitations

Limited degrees of freedom of instrument movement: Currently available laparoscopic instruments offer only 4 degrees of freedom of movement, i.e. rotation, up/down, left/right angulations; in/out movement for straight long instruments and 6 degrees of movements for curved instruments. This limitation has been overcome by new instruments available for Robotic surgery which have more degrees of movement. In contrast, in open surgery there are 360° of freedom of movement of instruments.

The limited degrees of freedom of movement make tissue handling with laparoscopic instruments more difficult. This is compounded with fixed position of entry ports. Instrument changes during laparoscopic surgery are more laborious and distracting. Port sites can be changed, and an experienced team will have no difficulty in changing instruments.

Less efficient instruments: A typical laparoscopic instrument transmits the force of a surgeon's hand from its handle to tip in ratio of only 3:1 in contrast to 1:3 ratio with a hemostat. The surgeon's hand therefore works about 6 times as hard to complete the same grasping task with the laparoscopic instrument. This is rarely a problem, and can be balanced by the fact that massively less retraction is required in awkward places.

Tactile feedback: There is a loss of direct tactile feedback because there is no direct contact of fingers with tissues. Indirect tactile feed back through instruments is markedly reduced due to the long length of instruments and because of friction between ports and instruments. This loss of indirect tactile feedback can lead to damage to tissue which has been grasped in an instrument, because the force which is being applied to grasped tissue is poorly appreciated by the surgeon's hand. This is only the case for a novice laparoscopic surgeon, and as the experience of the surgeon increases, the problem diminishes. Hand assisted minimal access surgery does not have this drawback.

Dark room: Operating room lights are turned off during laparoscopic surgery and the operating team works in relative darkness. Dark operating rooms during laparoscopic surgery increase the risk of collision hazards and using the wrong instruments. This can be overcome by providing a separate head light over the instrument trolley.

More clutter: The amount of equipment, tubes and cables is greater during laparoscopic surgery in comparison to open surgery. This creates a hazard for traffic movement. Multiple tubes and cables may create a jungle of connections in the operating field if not well organized. This may decrease the efficiency of instrument handling, positioning and exchanges. In a well laid out modern theater there are neatly laid cables to the laparoscopic stack, and the only extra cables to the patient are the light cable and video lead.

Tissue retrieval: Small port size limits the retrieval of solid, or bulky organs, and sometimes a small separate incision needs to be made in order to remove, for example, colon. For solid organs a morcellator can be used, or tissue can be broken up into small pieces by finger fracture. These methods may risk wound contamination, or tumor cell implantation at port sites during retrieval. The risks are however low, and port site tumor recurrence should not occur if good surgical techniques are adhered to.

Skills to Overcome Visual Limitations

Two dimensional imaging: Standard monitors in current use are two dimensional imaging systems. The surgeon has to reconstruct three dimensional pictures in his brain from the two dimensional output. This includes intense perceptual and mental processing, which continues throughout a laparoscopic procedure.

Limited view: There is a reduced field of vision and there is a decrease in the sensory input from the periphery of the field. There can be incidental tissue injury, when the instruments move outside the field of view. Movement of instruments within the abdomen must take place under direct vision to avoid accidental injury. This limitation is partly counterbalanced by the fact that the view is greatly magnified, and instruments can move anywhere in the abdominal cavity with ease.

Decoupling of the motor and visual spaces: Monitors should be placed in such a way that the visual axis formed between the surgeon's eyes and the monitor should be aligned with the hands and

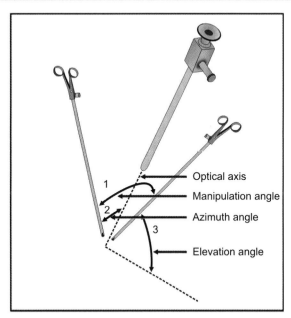

Fig. 10.1: Various angles (1) manipulation angle (2) Azimuth angle (3) Elevation angle

instruments. If they are not aligned it leads to poor task performance.

Port placement (Fig. 10.1): Proper placement is extremely important for successful completion of a laparoscopic procedure. Manipulation angle, Azimuth angle and Elevation angles guides the site for optimal port placement.

Manipulation Angle

This is the angle between the active and assisting instrument. Manipulation angle should be between 45 and 75° with the ideal angle being 60° for an efficient performance of intracorporeal knotting.

Azimuth Angle

This is the angle between either of the instruments and the optical axis of the endoscope. Better work efficiency is obtained with equal Azimuth angles.

Wide Azimuth angles should be avoided as far as possible.

Elevation Angle

This is the angle between the instrument and horizontal plane. Ideally the elevation angle should be equal to the manipulation angle.

Ports should be placed in such a way that the ratio of intracorporeal and extracorporeal length of instrument should be 2:1.

Ports for instruments and endoscope should be placed in such a way that instrument and endoscope are aligned in the same direction. One should not operate against the camera, because the surgeon will be working on a mirror image and manipulations become difficult in that situation.

Monitor Location

The monitor should ideally be placed in front of the surgeon and below eye level range (0 to 45°, 25° ideal) in order to produce a gaze down view. Gaze down viewing permits sensory signals and motor control to have a closed spatial location and being visual signals in correspondence with instrument manipulations. The design of laparoscopic stacks is such that the monitors are usually at eye level.

Principles of Camera Operation

The camera operator's role is crucial in laparoscopic surgery because the camera is the eye of surgeon and surgeon will only see those things shown by the camera. The camera operator actively takes part in surgery.

Golden Rules for Camera Operation

1. Keep the task in the center of the field, which has best illumination and least image distortion, so that the surgeon sees the best quality image. Another reason for keeping in the center is that if the surgeon works in the periphery of the field, instrument movement may take place outside the displayed image, and can accidentally damage adjacent structures.

2. If the surgeon wants better resolution of the target area for doing fine work, e.g. dissection or picking up a fallen clip, advance the telescope towards the target area, which will increase the resolution but decrease the size of visual field. During insertion of instruments or knot tying, a wider visual field is required and the laparoscope should be kept away from target area. When the surgeon becomes more experienced this may not be necessary.

3. Avoid jerky movements because they hinder precise surgery.

4. Keep the camera oriented at all times with a level horizon.

5. Before starting the procedure, do a white balancing of the camera and focus the camera on a gauze swab on the drapes.

6. During port insertion, keep the portion of the abdomen where the port will enter in the centre of the monitor field at all times to avoid injury to intra-abdominal organs.

7. During instrument insertion, the camera holder should guide the surgeon by showing a panoramic view for proper insertion of instruments. This becomes less important with a more experienced surgeon.

Selection of Laparoscope (Fig. 10.2)

Each endoscope has an optical axis and a physical axis. The optical axis is the axis passing through the center of the visual field of the laparoscope. The physical axis is the axis passing through the center of the endoscope. The endoscope can be 0°, 30° or 45° depending on the angle between optical axis and physical axis. The 30° laparoscope is useful in pelvic surgery and for difficult cholecystectomy. The 45° laparoscope is used for bariatric

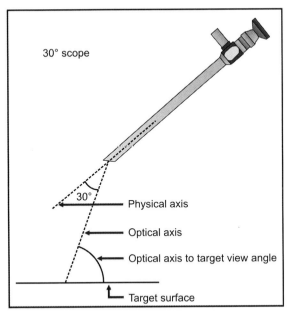

30° scope

30°

Physical axis

Optical axis

Optical axis to target view angle

Target surface

Fig. 10.2: Physical axis and optical axis of a telescope

surgery. For common procedures a 0° laparoscope is sufficient.

Camera angles can be changed during procedure by passing it through different ports thus improving the field of vision.

Basic Requirements for Laparoscopic Surgery

Important basic equipment for laparoscopic surgery includes:
1. A rapid-flow insufflator
2. A light source
3. Video camera and camera cable
4. A laparoscope
5. At least one monitor
6. Electrosurgical unit
7. Suction-irrigation machine
8. Laparoscopic instruments and ports.

The Rapid-Flow Insufflator

Carbon dioxide (CO_2) is used to create a pneumoperitoneum, creating a working space by distending the anterior, and lateral abdominal walls.

CO_2 is preferred because:

It is an inert gas, and does not support combustion.

It is highly soluble, easily absorbed into the blood and easily excreted by the lungs.

It is readily available, inexpensive and non-toxic.

Automatic insufflators are used for insufflation of gas. These have a sensor, which can deliver a preset pressure of CO_2 and can control intra-abdominal pressure and rate of flow. Flow rate will increase if the intra-abdominal pressure falls below a preset level and flow rate automatically stops once the preset intra-abdominal pressure is reached.

Modern automatic insufflators have bacteriological filters which can be incorporated along gas lines and can increase the temperature of the gas up to 37°, to prevent hypothermia during long laparoscopic procedures.

Physiology of Carbon Dioxide Pneumoperitoneum

CO_2 instilled into peritoneal cavity normally diffuses across the peritoneal surface into the venous circulation. After CO_2 is carried away by the venous system, it can be eliminated by the lungs or stored elsewhere in the body. The human body can store up to 120 liters of CO_2 and bone is the largest potential long term reservoir. Skeletal muscles and other potential visceral stores come into play if retention occurs for less than an hour. After storage, CO_2 is mainly eliminated by the lungs. Following a long laparoscopic procedure, it might take several hours for the accumulated CO_2 to be eliminated and for the body's acid base balance to be restored to normal.

Pathophysiology of Pneumoperitoneum

Effects of CO_2

a. Direct local effects
b. Centrally mediated effects.

Direct local effects:
1. Decreased cardiac contractility
2. Pulmonary hypertension
3. Systemic vasodilatation

Centrally mediated effects:

Hypercarbia leads to widespread sympathetic stimulation:

a. Tachycardia
b. Vasoconstriction
c. Increased central venous pressure
d. Increased mean arterial pressure
e. Increased pulmonary artery pressure and pulmonary vascular resistance.

Volume Effects of Pneumoperitoneum

1. Elevation of diaphragm, and anterolateral abdominal wall.
2. Decreased venous return due to increased pressure on the inferior vena cava.

Physiological Effects of Elevation of Diaphragm

1. Decreased functional residual capacity
2. Increased ventilation-perfusion mismatch
3. Increased intrapulmonary shunting
4. Increased alveolar-arterial gradient of oxygen partial pressure.

These effects are overcome by increasing the mechanical ventilation rate and concentration of inspired oxygen.

Physiological Effects of Decreased Venous Return

1. Initial increase in cardiac index followed by
2. Cardiac index decrease (20-59%)
3. Cardiac axis of the heart shifts causing electro-cardiography alteration
4. 65% increase in systemic resistance
5. 90% increase in pulmonary vascular resistance.

These effects are overcome by an adequate volume load.

Neuro-endocrine and Metabolic Changes after Pneumoperitoneum

1. Four fold increase of renin and aldosterone
2. Release of vasopressin, adrenaline and nor-adrenaline leading to sympathetic mimetic response
3. Renal vasoconstriction leading to urinary sodium retention and temporary tubular renal dysfunction
4. Hypothermia due to escape of water vapor along with gas leakage. Water vapor takes latent heat of vaporization along with it causing heat loss. It is just like a wind blowing over the exposed abdominal contents. In a prolonged procedure, core temperature can drop and hypothermia may result.

Light Sources

Light sources commonly in use are:
1. Xenon
2. Metal halide
3. Halogen.

Both Xenon and metal halide give natural white light but the light of a xenon source is more natural. Halogen gives a yellow light, which is compensated by white balancing in the video camera system. All modern light sources have infrared filters. Commercially available xenon light sources can give an intensity varying from 150-300W. They have automatic intensity control which gives continuous optical illumination. Light from the source is carried to the laparoscope by a flexible light cable and down the laparoscope by a solid lens.

Light cables can be made up of:
1. Glass fiber light cable
2. Special fluid filled cable.

Glass fiber light cables are more flexible but less efficient than fluid light cables because of fiber mismatch at the source or fibre breakage. Glass fiber light cables can be autoclaved but fluid filled ones cannot.

Precautions to be taken during Handling of Light Source and Cable

1. The light source should not be shone directly into the eye when unplugged from the laparoscope, as the very high intensity can cause retinal damage.
2. The ends of light cables can become very hot, with temperatures reaching up to 95°C, with the possibility of burns to anyone handling it. To prevent injury, the light source should initially be set on its lowest level (10-25%), and should be switched off when laparoscope is not in use. Light sources should have a fan to prevent the temperature rising too high and also to increase the life of the expensive bulbs.

Video Cameras

The cameras used in laparoscopy are miniature cameras based on a charged couple device (CCD). Chip camera systems have two components:
1. The camera head attached to the laparoscope.
2. The camera controller unit, which is located on an adjacent trolley which usually also holds the insufflator, and a monitor.

The camera head consists of an objective lens and CCD chip. The lens focuses the image onto a CCD chip. The chip converts incoming photons into electronic charges and produces picture elements (pixels). This is possible because CCD chip is covered by a layer of light sensitive photoreceptors. The signal is then transmitted to the camera processing unit, where the image is generated for the monitor.

There are two types of cameras, single chip and three chip. In the single chip camera, only one chip processes all three primary colours. In three chip cameras, there is a separate chip for each primary colour, i.e. red, green, and blue. This improves image definition.

Creating a Safe Pneumoperitoneum

There are two main methods of creating a safe pneumoperitoneum:
1. The closed method
2. The open method.

The Closed Method

A Verres needle is used to create a pneumoperitoneum. The Verres needle is a hollow needle with a spring loaded blunt centre core. The proximal end has a Luer lock which may be closed with a tap. The patency of the needle and spring loaded mechanism should be tested before using it.

The umbilicus is usually used for insertion of the Verres needle but in very obese patients or in patients with a history of previous abdominal surgery, the left or right hypochondrium midclavicular line can be used.

In both areas, the needle should be held like a pen and directed towards the pelvic cavity rather than vertically downwards. Often, two "clicks" can be felt as the needle penetrates the abdominal wall, and the blunt trochar springs forward, firstly through muscle or linea alba, then again through peritoneum. It is necessary to ascertain the safe position of the needle in the peritoneal cavity following insertion.

The following tests are performed to make sure the Verres needle is in a safe position.
1. Attach a syringe to the Verres needle and aspirate. If intestinal contents or blood are aspirated, the needle should be withdrawn, as bowel or vascular injury may have occurred. In practice this happens rarely.

2. *The saline drop test*: A drop of saline put over the hub of the needle with the Luer lock opened, should be sucked inside the peritoneal cavity because of negative pressure. Saline should flow freely into the needle without difficulty.

3. Initial slow insufflation of CO_2 at a rate of one liter per minute should produce an initial intra-abdominal pressure of 5-7 mmHg. If the initial pressure reading is above 10 mmHg, the needle may be lying in the pre-peritoneal space, mesentery, or omentum.

Once a safe pneumoperitoneum has been created, the first port insertion is usually via the umbilicus, directed towards the coccyx, preferably with a retractable blade to minimise the possibility of visceral damage.

In a variation of this technique, the laparoscope can be placed down the center of a different sort of port (Optiview, Visiport), with a transparent blunt tip, enabling the operator to see the tissues splitting, and the peritoneum opening *under vision*.

The Open Method (Fig. 10.3)

A vertical or horizontal 2 cm long infraumbilical incision is made. The incision is deepened down to the linea Alba.

The linear Alba is incised between stay sutures and peritoneum is exposed, and then incised for 1 cm *under vision*.

A finger is inserted inside peritoneal cavity to sweep away any adhesions, and a blunt tipped trocar is then inserted *under vision*. Stay sutures can be used to secure the port.

Due to the size of the initial incision, gas leakage around the initial port can occur. A gas proof seal can be obtained by putting stitches around the port into skin over paraffin gauze, or a special port with occlusive balloons at the tip, known as a Hasson's cannula can be used. The port has to be closed and repaired carefully at the end of the procedure, to prevent port site hernias developing.

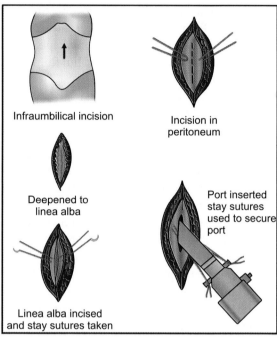

Infraumbilical incision

Incision in peritoneum

Deepened to linea alba

Port inserted stay sutures used to secure port

Linea alba incised and stay sutures taken

Fig. 10.3: Various steps for inserting first port by open method

The open method is now the most commonly taught technique, as it has a lower incidence of bowel and vascular injury. It is not used universally, however, as the closed method is quicker, and produces a smaller scar. The serious vascular injury rate for the closed technique is in the range of 1:1000 insertions.

Summary of ergonomic physical recommendations for optimizing the working conditions in laparoscopic surgery:

1. Foot pedal should be near the foot and at the same level.

2. Instrument handle should be at or slightly below elbow height.

3. Shoulders should be relaxed and arms should not be elevated.

4. There should be proper choice of instrument handle and grasp configuration for each task

KEY POINTS

1. Minimal access surgery is not always minimally invasive.
2. Proper selection of equipment and proper training is necessary before one embarks upon laparoscopic surgery.
3. Proper placement of ports is the key to success of laparoscopic surgery.
4. Safe creation of pneumoperitoneum is of paramount importance for starting of any laparoscopic procedure.
5. Open method for creation of pneumoperitoneum is safer than closed method with zero incidences of vascular injuries and a very low incidence of gut injuries.
6. There are mechanical and visual limitations of laparoscopic surgery which can be overcome by experience.
7. If intracorporeal suturing is planned, the manipulation angle between active instrument and assisting instrument should be 45°.

Hemostasis

The ability to control bleeding is an essential surgical skill which every surgeon must acquire. It is important that during an episode of hemorrhage the surgeon should maintain his or her composure and control bleeding without causing damage to surrounding structures. One should always ask for senior help if one is not able to control bleeding.

Types of Bleeding

According to source:
1. *Arterial* bleeding is bright red, pulsatile, comes under pressure and is brisk.
2. *Venous* bleeding is dark red, continuous, low pressure, non-pulsatile, and difficult to control in comparison to arterial bleeding.
3. *Capillary* bleeding is constant slow ooze from a raw area. It can usually be controlled by pressure.

According to Time of Bleeding

1. *Primary hemorrhage* is bleeding that occurs at the time of surgery or as a result of trauma. Bleeding may be excessive if there is an altered bleeding or clotting profile, e.g. liver disease, obstructive jaundice, malnutrition, hemophilia or if there is disease of arteries which prevent constriction of blood vessels, e.g. atherosclerosis.
2. *Reactionary hemorrhage* occurs within 24 hours of an operation. It usually occurs from small

blood vessels on raw surfaces or from a minor capsular laceration or from a suture or staple line of anastomosis. Reactionary bleeding is usually caused by a rise in arterial or venous pressure leading to dislodgement of clots. This may be caused by pain, or excessive straining.

Reactionary hemorrhage can occur after laparoscopic surgery, when small blood vessels compressed by increased intra-abdominal pressure start bleeding when the pneumoperitoneum is desufflated. Careful hemostasis is of paramount importance to avoid this problem.

3. *Secondary hemorrhage* usually occurs 7-10 days after surgery. It is usually due to an infection such as β hemolytic streptococci cause dissolution of blood clots. Examples of secondary bleeding include bleeding from tonsil bed after tonsillectomy, bleeding from an infected area after biliary surgery or bleeding from infected vascular grafts. This type of hemorrhage may be secondary to auto digestion of blood clot following pancreatic surgery.

Bleeding during Surgery

During surgery some bleeding is inevitable. Blood loss tends to be greater during long or complex procedures such as liver resection, esophageal resection, and major joint surgery. Every surgeon must acquire the skills necessary to firstly minimize blood loss, and secondly control hemorrhage during surgery.

Prevention

1. In certain diseases such as obstructive jaundice, malnutrition, chronic liver disease and in hemophilia patients there is an increased propensity to bleed. In these situations the bleeding and clotting profiles should be brought to normal. In obstructive jaundice and chronic liver disease intramuscular administration of 10 mg vitamin K often brings the prothrombin time to normal. In cases of emergency surgery, infusion of fresh frozen plasma often replenishes the deficient clotting factors.

2. If the patient is on oral anticoagulants, or heparin, these should be stopped before surgery and the coagulation profile should be brought back to normal. Aspirin should ideally be stopped one week before surgery.

3. Blood transfusion service protocols should be checked in order to decide if a blood sample is to be "Grouped and Saved", or if blood is to be cross matched. The availability of cross matched blood should be checked prior to surgery.

4. The technique of hypotensive anesthesia may help minimize blood loss.

5. During head and neck surgery, raising the head of the table 15-20° reduces venous congestion and blood loss.

6. While raising skin flaps during thyroid or breast surgery blood loss can be reduced by infiltration of normal saline or normal saline mixed with adrenaline (1: 200,000). Fluid raises the tissue pressure, renders tissue transparent, and opens up the plane of dissection. Adrenaline produces local vasoconstriction.

7. Revise the anatomy before starting any major surgery. This helps in identification of major blood vessels before they are injured.

8. If you are operating upon blood vessels or major organs, control of inflow vessels often helps in reducing bleeding. Non-crushing vascular clamps can be applied across the pedicle of an organ or the pedicle can be encircled with a tape prior to dissection.

9. If operating upon huge vascular tumors, preoperative embolization of feeding vessels might reduce intra-operative bleeding, provided surgery is performed within 48-72 hours of embolisation. After 48 hours, there is development of neo-vessels which make surgery more difficult.

10. The tourniquet is a commonly used method for reducing blood loss when operating upon limbs. It is contraindicated in the presence of chronic ischemia, impending gangrene, and spreading cellulitis or in the presence of bony fractures.

Before applying a tourniquet, the limb is emptied of blood by elevating it for 2-3 minutes. A pneumatic tourniquet is applied on the proximal part of the limb over orthopedic wool. An Esmarch's bandage can be applied over the limb for more complete exsanguination, but it must be applied before applying the tourniquet. It too is contraindicated in the presence of cellulitis.

A tourniquet is applied around the upper arm or upper thigh over a thin layer of orthopedic wool and is inflated to 70-100 mmHg above systolic pressure (200 mmHg for arm and around 300 mmHg for a leg. It should be released after every 2 hours for 10 minutes before reapplying it.

Control of Hemorrhage

1. *Manual pressure* by packing or by a metal retractor over a pack is an invaluable method for control of bleeding. It is the method of choice for control of generalized oozing. Packing

should be immediately employed whenever there is a substantial bleeding especially in a deep cavity or other inaccessible area. Manual compression should be exerted over packs for 5 minutes observed by the theatre clock. This maneuver provides immediate control, and the surgeon then has time to prepare himself for any necessary further action. Packing alone may be sufficient for certain clinical situations, e.g. extensive liver injuries. It also provides an opportunity for the anaesthetist to stabilize the patient.

Manual pressure may occasionally be employed during laparoscopic surgery by using an atraumatic instrument or adjacent tissue over the bleeding area.

2. *Clips and simple ligatures* are commonly used methods of securing haemostasis. Vessels of 2 to 5 mm in diameter can be occluded by clips or simple ligatures. While applying a clip one should make sure that it surrounds the vessel completely. The clip should make an angle of 90 degrees with the long axis of the vessel which should then be divided 3-4 millimeters away from the clip or ligature, to prevent slippage. Clips and ligatures should not be too tightly applied, because it can lead to weakness of the vessel wall by the cheese-wire cutting effect, especially in cases of rigid, non-elastic arteries due to atherosclerosis in older patients.

3. *Energized systems*: The following devices can be used for thermal coagulation and sealing of blood vessels.
a. Electrocoagulation
b. Ultrasonic sealing
c. Ligasure sealing
d. Photocoagulation.

Electrocoagulation is safe for sealing of vessels up to 2 mm. Ultrasonic sealing is used for sealing of vessels up to 5 mm. Ultrasonic sealing uses mechanical waves not audible by the human ear, i.e. frequency more than 20000 cycles per second. These waves propagate in matter but not in air. These waves impart power density that is less than electrocautery or laser. They cause less tissue heating with reduced penetration. These machines generate waves between 20-60 kHz frequencies produced by piezoelectric transducer. They can cut, coagulate or separate tissue by high power density of around 100 W per second. The Ligasure is used for sealing of vessels up to 7 mm.

4. *Transfixion and double ligature*: If an arterial stump continues to pulsate after simple ligature, this may indicate that the ligature is not safe and may fail due to the force of transmitted pulsation. Such a stump should be made safe by a transfixion stitch, in which either 2-0 or 3-0 vicryl on a round bodied needle is passed through the wall of the stump, and tied on one side, then encircling the stump, and tied firmly on the other side with a surgeon's knot. Transfixion prevents the displacement of ligature. Transfixion and double ligature is generally needed for vessels over 5 mm in diameter, such as the femoral artery, splenic artery or renal artery.

An experienced surgeon will often use a transfixion stitch on a large artery as a safety measure prior to division, during an elective procedure.

5. *Suturing of stump*: Suturing of a proximal arterial stump is still occasionally performed, using a prolene stitch.

6. *Vascular stapler*: This instrument (EndoGIA) can be used to provide a simple and safe way of dividing vascular pedicles laparoscopically. It may also be used in inaccessible areas at open surgery. The instrument fires two rows of vascular staples across the artery, and then cuts between the two staple lines. It is quick, effective, and very expensive.

Things to do After Control of Hemorrhage

1. Do not close up immediately, but wait until the patient is stabilized, so that you can identify any other areas of bleeding which may not have declared themselves due to hypotension.
2. One should wash out blood from body cavities with saline. Blood left inside a cavity can act as a nidus for bacterial proliferation and the patient may also develop icterus in the post operative period due to absorption of products of broken down hemoglobin.
3. Before closure, always make sure that you have not caused damage to other vital structures, e.g. damage to the common bile duct while controlling bleeding from a cystic artery.

KEY POINTS

1. Every surgeon must be able to control hemorrhage during surgery.
2. In cases of unexpected bleeding keep cool and composed.
3. Pack the bleeding area to buy time and organize yourself.
4. Inform anesthesiologist.
5. Do not hesitate to ask for senior's help if you are not confident.
6. Wait for ten minutes before removing pack.
7. By this time bleeding will often have reduced to a trickle to identify the bleeding point.
8. If packing does not help, proximal and distal control of a vessel may be needed.
9. If there is bleeding from great vessel, suturing of a tear in the vessel may be required.

Biopsy Techniques

Biopsy is a process in which tissue is obtained for microscopic or other investigations. It is not analogous to fine needle aspiration, which obtains only cells. Fine needle aspiration is an alternative to biopsy but not a substitute, as there are many clinical situations in which there is no alternative to biopsy. Details of histological architecture and immunohistochemistry are only obtainable from biopsy specimens.

Indications for Biopsy

1. To confirm the diagnosis of malignancy, when there is strong clinical suspicion but repeated fine needle aspiration is not conclusive or is negative.
2. In suspected cases of soft tissue sarcoma, lymphoma or follicular carcinoma of thyroid. In these cases fine needle aspiration cannot establish an exact diagnosis.
3. To differentiate between primary malignancy and metastasis.
4. In cases of breast malignancy where estrogen receptor status is required.
5. To differentiate between *in situ* carcinoma and invasive carcinoma.
6. Sub typing of malignancy for staging and prognostication.
7. In cases of testicular malignancy, if there are residual retroperitoneal masses postradiotherapy or chemotherapy. Excision biopsy is necessary to differentiate between residual malignancy and fibrosis.

8. Tissue is mandatory if any disease requires investigation with electron microscopy, enzyme histochemistry, and immunohistochemistry.

Enzyme histochemistry is required:
1. For diagnosis of myopathies,
2. For diagnosis of malabsorption and alactasia,
3. For Hirschsprung's disease.

Immunohistochemistry is needed
1. For typing of lymphoid tumors,
2. For identification of germ cell tumors (placental alkaline phosphatase),
3. Melanoma (by S-100, HMB45 and Vimetin),
4. Thyroid tumor (by thyroglobulin),
5. Vascular tumor (Endothelial marker, e.g. Factor VIII),
6. For identification of soft tissue tumors.
   The objective of a tissue biopsy is to obtain a tissue sample
1. Which is representative of the pathology.
2. With preserved tissue architecture.
3. Which includes a portion of normal tissue for comparison.

Rules of Tissue Biopsy

1. In a large lesion there can be areas of normal tissue in between lesions or there can be heterogeneity. To avoid sampling errors one should take multiple biopsies from different places.

2. In an ulcerated or fungating lesion, biopsy should not be taken from the centre, because this will most probably show necrotic tissue. Always take a biopsy from the periphery of the lesion, including normal tissue with it.
3. If it is surgically feasible and safe for the patient, always include the full thickness of the lesion in a biopsy to assess the depth of the lesion. This is especially important in staging of malignant melanoma.
4. Deeply situated masses may be surrounded by compressed normal surrounding tissue, forming a pseudocapsule. One should make sure that the biopsy traverses through this normal tissue in to the actual site of pathology before obtaining tissue. Failure to do so might result in a false negative report.
5. Avoid handling biopsy tissue with crushing forceps or traumatic instruments, because this will lead to loss of tissue architecture, which is especially important in diagnosis of lymphoma.
6. Do not use laser or the cryoprobe whilst obtaining a biopsy, as they destroy ttissue.
7. Do not use a morcellator for retrieving a solid organ after laparoscopic surgery, if you want a tissue diagnosis postoperatively.
8. Orientation of the resected specimen is important, if you need information on tumor free resected margins or staging. Orientation should be carried out in theater by pinning out, or labeling with colored sutures.

Types of Biopsy

1. Open biopsy
2. Percutaneous closed biopsy
3. Endoscopic biopsy
4. Laparoscopic biopsy

Open Biopsy

Open biopsy is usually performed for lesions in the skin and subcutaneous tissues. It is now unusual to open the abdomen or chest just for the sake of obtaining tissue.

Types of open biopsy
a. *Shave biopsy*: A scalpel or razor is used to shave off a thin layer of the lesion parallel to the skin.
b. *Punch biopsy*: A small cylindrical punch is screwed in to the lesion through full thickness and a cylinder of tissue is removed. One to two stitches may be needed to close the wound.
c. *Incision biopsy*: Incision biopsy involves removal of a wedge of the lesion with adjacent normal tissue. Incision biopsy is used for large lesions prior to treatment.
d. *Excision biopsy*: In this entire lesion is excised with a surrounding rim of normal tissue. This used for small lesions, which can be excised completely.

Percutaneous closed biopsy can be:
1. Image guided
2. Blind

Image guided percutaneous biopsy is the method of choice, usually reserved for deep seated inaccessible lesions. Image guidance can be through ultrasonography or CT, and with the help of either it is usually feasible to find a safe path or window through which the biopsy needle can pass into the region of interest.

Blind Biopsy

This can be used for superficial palpable lesions, kidney, liver and prostate. Various types of needles may be used.
1. Abraham's needle for pleural biopsy
2. Menghini needle for liver biopsy
3. Trucut needle
4. Automatic, spring loaded modification of Trucut needle (Fig. 12.1).
5. High speed drill biopsy for bone only.

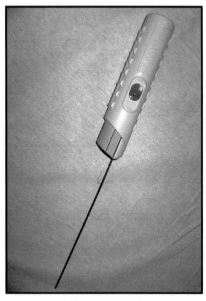

Fig. 12.1: Trucut needle

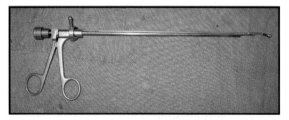

Fig. 12.2: Cystoscopic biopsy forcep

Endoscopic Biopsy (Fig. 12.2)

This can be used in association with both rigid and flexible endoscopy. Varieties of biopsy forceps are available. Since these biopsy forceps remove a very small amount of tissue, multiple biopsies at different points may need to be taken.

Post-biopsy Procedure

1. A proper histology request form must be completed. Every specimen must be labelled correctly. The form must contain the patient's identification details, nature of specimen, clinical features, operative details and presumptive diagnosis. Patient details on the request form should match with the label on the specimen jar or container. Pathologists will also need to know if the patient had neo-adjuvant chemotherapy for a full pathological staging report.

2. The specimen should be put in the appropriate fixative. Ten percent buffered formalin is suitable for most specimens.

Frozen Section

This is a special technique in which tissue is sent fresh to the pathology department, where it is frozen to $-25°C$ using either liquid nitrogen or CO_2. After freezing, the tissue is immediately sectioned using a microtome in a special chamber known as a cryostat. Cut frozen sections are stained with Hemotoxylin and Eosin for immediate reporting. There has to be good coordination between the surgical and pathology teams when using this technique. Frozen sections are more difficult to interpret than ordinary paraffin sections and the services of an experienced pathologist are needed. It can be a highly accurate technique with false negative rates of 0.5% and a false positive rate of 0.1%.

Role of Frozen Section in Modern Day Clinical Practice

1. To establish the benign or malignant nature of a lesion during surgery, in order to decide on the extent of a resection. An example of this would be the management of solitary nodular goiter with fine needle aspiration report of follicular pathology. In this situation the surgeon may perform a lobectomy and send it for frozen section. If the report is follicular carcinoma, he completes the procedure by doing a near total thyroidectomy. If the report is follicular adenoma, lobectomy itself is sufficient.

2. To ensure that resected margins are tumor free in malignancy. One of the example is breast conservation surgery, in which the surgeon can revise the resected margins if not tumor free.

3. To establish that a biopsy contains sufficient material for diagnosis and is from a representative area in a difficult case.

Precautions to be taken during Special Situations

Biopsy of an impalpable breast lesion detected by breast screening:

1. Preoperative X-ray localization and insertion of localizing needle under X-ray control, by the radiologist in a radiology suite is performed.
2. Suspected lesion with localizing needle is removed.
3. Removed specimen along with needle is X-rayed and compared with preoperative mammogram film.
4. If image of removed specimen does not match with abnormality on mammogram, more tissue is removed.
5. Boundaries of removed specimen are marked with dye.
6. Removed specimen in sliced into serial 5 mm thickness sections on a special X-ray board and image again taken to determine which sections contain the exact lesion, which can then be further processed.

Lymph Node Biopsy

Which Lymph Node should be Removed?

1. If there are involved lymph nodes in different anatomical areas, then choose an area which is more likely to be involved in the suspected pathology. For example in a suspected case of Hodgkin's lymphoma with involvement of cervical, axillary and inguinal lymph node, biopsy from an axillary lymph node will be preferred to that of a cervical or inguinal one.
2. If there are multiple lymph nodes in one anatomical group, then choose a lymph node which is least likely to be involved in non-specific infection. Example is cervical lymphadenitis with involvement of submental, submandibular and posterior cervical lymph nodes. In this clinical situation, biopsy from a posterior cervical group of lymph nodes is a more sensible choice because lymph nodes of submental and submandibular region are commonly involved in non specific infections of throat.

3. Choose a lymph node for biopsy which does not overlie and underlie an important structure. Excision biopsy is preferred over incision biopsy.
4. After biopsy the lymph node is bisected to inspect for gross pathology, i.e. caseous material, stony hard lymph node or lymph node containing pus. On bisection, imprints are taken on glass slides and stained. One half of the lymph node is sent in formalin for H and E staining. Remaining half is divided in to three parts. One piece is fixed in glutaraldehyde for electron microscopy.

Another piece is snap frozen to –70°C for enzyme and immunohistochemistry. If infective pathology, e.g. tuberculosis is suspected, then remaining piece is kept in saline and stored at 4°C for microbiological examination.

KEY POINTS

1. In spite of advances in cytology techniques, biopsy techniques have a definite role.
2. Taking a biopsy is a basic surgical skill which surgeon must acquire.
3. Tissue for biopsy must be taken from representative area of pathology.
4. Excision biopsy is preferable to incision biopsy.
5. Avoid taking a biopsy from the center of an ulcerating tumor.
6. Always include a portion of normal tissue while taking a biopsy from an ulcer.
7. Core needle biopsy is a good alternative to incision biopsy.
8. Always properly label biopsy specimens and give adequate details of clinical history and operative procedure to help the pathologist.
9. Send a biopsy specimen in the proper solution according to need.
10. If planning for frozen section inform pathologist well in advance.

Dissection Techniques

DISSECTION

Dissection is an essential component for the successful completion of any surgical procedure. Quality of dissection is often judged as the hallmark of surgical competence. The technique of surgical dissection can be mastered by adopting sound surgical principals as well as by familiarity with surgical anatomy.

DEFINITION

Dissection is a latin word derived from (dis = apart + secare = to cut). It can be defined as "the exposure of a target organ or area by the process of separation of overlying tissue with hemostasis and preservation of surrounding essential or vital structures".

A good dissection requires not only a through knowledge of anatomy, but also a good understanding of the pathology of the relevant area.

Components of Dissection

1. Sensory component comprising of visual and tactile elements.
2. Access component involving tissue manipulation and instrument maneuvers.

The end point of good dissection is exposure of the target structure so that the desired procedure can be performed upon it.

Prerequisite of a Good Dissection

1. Application of the right amount of stretch on the tissues (without trauma) before starting to

dissect. This entirely depends upon tactile feedback which the surgeon acquires during the initial years of training. Tension or stretching of tissues in the correct direction helps in identification of attachments and natural planes of separation.
2. Identification of proper tissue planes.
3. Economy of movement. Each and every action the surgeon takes should be productive and should help in achieving the desired objective. Unproductive actions increase the chances of complications, and lead to fatigue. The surgeon should complete one step of the operation before proceeding to the next step.

Modes of Dissection

Available modes of dissection are as follows:
1. Blunt dissection
2. Sharp scissor or scalpel dissection
3. Ultrasonic dissection
4. Dissection by electrocautery
5. Hydrodissection by high velocity and high pressure water
6. Dissection by Laser
7. Radiofrequency ablation.

Blunt Dissection

Blunt dissection is suitable in places where there is a good amount of loose areolar tissue which can be separated by application of shear force. The safety of blunt dissection depends upon the sensitivity of tactile feedback to the surgeon's hands, which can differentiate between important structures, e.g. vessels or nerves and areolar tissue. Blunt dissection is especially useful in area where anatomy is obscured.

Techniques of Blunt Dissection

1. Separation or splitting of overlying tissue. This is especially useful while dissecting along tubular structures such as vessels, nerves or ureter.
2. Tearing or teasing
3. Wiping
4. Distraction
5. Peeling.

Methods of Blunt Dissection

1. *Finger dissection*: A tearing or shearing action can be performed by a finger along the line of separation. The tip of the finger can be used to peel off a structure, e.g. separation of gall-bladder from its bed during cholecystectomy. Sometimes blunt dissection is performed by gauze wrapped on a finger, e.g. dissection of a hernial sac from the cord structures during inguinal hernia repair. Finger fracture technique may be used for liver resection.
2. *Peeling* action can also be performed by a pledget of gauze held in a forcep to peel off fibrous tissue. During cholecystectomy, dissection in Calot's triangle is very often performed using this method.
3. *Closed scissor tips* can be used as blunt dissectors. This technique is commonly used during lysis of adhesions during laparotomy.
4. *Splitting action* is often performed by scissor points to separate muscle fibres without cutting them, e.g. splitting of internal oblique/transversus abdominis muscle during appendicectomy.
5. *Right angle forcep* or Maryland dissector is commonly used for blunt dissection behind

vascular bundles. It can, however, split, peel off or tear underlying structures, and therefore needs to be used with care.
6. *Suction cannula* is sometimes used as blunt dissection especially during laparoscopic surgery, often in conjunction with hydro-dissection.

Sharp Dissection

Sharp dissection involves division of tissues by cutting performed by a scalpel or by scissors. Sharp dissection is a two handed procedure and needs application of the desired amount of tension by the non-dominant hand with division and separation performed by the active hand. The technique of traction and counter-traction is often utilized whilst raising flaps during mastectomy or during thyroid surgery.

Diathermy Dissection

There are two types of handheld diathermy used commonly for dissection.
1. *Handheld disposable diathermy probe* with cutting and coagulation buttons. This is frequently used instead of scissors to divide tissues, and coagulate small vessels simultaneously. It facilitates a bloodless field, and has to be used carefully in the abdomen to avoid diathermy injury to bowel.
2. *Monopolar and bipolar scissors.* These are of the McIndoe variety, and come in various lengths for superficial or deep dissection. They combine the dissecting properties of McIndoe scissors with the properties of the handheld diathermy probe. They are particularly useful during abdominal and neck dissections. The diathermy works from a foot pedal and can be used selectively for tissues such as peritoneum, and serosa. They are useful for dividing adhesions. The bipolar scissors are safer to

use, as adjacent tissues cannot be damaged by diathermy. This is because the current passes between the two scissors blades. These scissors have a limited life as they cannot be sharpened, and have to be replaced after 20-30 uses.

Ultrasonic Dissection

Ultrasonic dissectors are of two types:
1. Low power system
2. High power system

The low power system (CUSA SELECTOR) is used for liver surgery. These systems cleave water containing tissues by cavitation leaving organized structures with low water content intact.

High power system, e.g. Autosonix, Harmonic Scalpel. This cleaves loose areolar tissue and blood vessels up to 3 mm diameter by fractional heating, performs coagulating and cutting action at the same time. It uses mechanical energy in the range of 55000 cycles/sec, and acts by disruption of hydrogen bonds and formation of a coagulum. It produces less heat in comparison to electrocautery and causes less collateral damage and tissue necrosis. The tip of the instrument remains very hot for several seconds after use, and caution needs to be taken to avoid it touching and burning adjacent tissues such as bowel, or the surgeon's fingers.

High Velocity Water Jet Dissection

This type of dissection disrupts friable, soft tissue but leaves ducts and blood vessels intact. It also has the effect of washing away adherent clot, which makes identification of anatomy much easier, for example in dissection of Calot's triangle.

Laser Dissection

A variety of lasers may be used in surgery for dissection. Laser light is used to heat a probe to white heat – for example a sapphire crystal. This very intense heat is very efficient at cutting dense fibrous tissue, and may help to produce an almost bloodless field. Lasers are very expensive, and need strict protocols to avoid the hazards of eye exposure in theatre. Training is required in their use in specialized situations. Types of laser used include CO_2 laser, Holmium laser, KTP laser, Nd YAG laser.

KEY POINTS

1. Dissection is an essential component for successful completion of any surgical procedure.
2. Quality of dissection is the hallmark of surgical competence.
3. Good dissection requires application of the right amount of stretch, identification of tissue planes and economy of movement.
4. Dissection can be either sharp or blunt.
5. Various devices like diathermy, ultrasonic machine or laser can be used for dissection.
6. Blunt dissection is useful in places where there is plenty of areolar tissue and anatomy is obscured.
7. Blunt dissection can be performed by finger, pledget of gauze held in a forceps, closed scissor tips, or by Maryland dissector.
8. Sharp dissection involves division of tissues by cutting using scissors or scalpel.

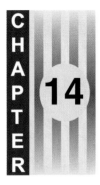

Surgical Diathermy: Principles and Precautions

CHAPTER 14

Diathermy was introduced during the early twentieth surgery by Cushing and Bovie. When ever an electrical current passes through our body it induces intense neuromuscular stimulation and alteration of cardiac rhythm. This effect was described by Michel Faraday. With the increase in the frequency of alternating current, neuromuscular stimulation decreases and disappears at 500000Hz (50KHz). Electrosurgery units work on the principal of converting normal frequency alternating current (50 Hz) to high frequency alternating current (50 KHz). Modern day electrosurgical units can produce currents in the range of 200-300 KHz. Neuromuscular stimulation does not occur at such frequencies because current changes direction so rapidly that ionic exchange at cellular level does not occur, and muscle is not stimulated. High frequency alternating current, when concentrated on a small area, however, produces very high temperatures, capable of coagulating tissues.

Uses of Diathermy

1. *For coagulation*

Three types of coagulation modes can be used:

a. Soft coagulation is the safest for both open and laparoscopic surgery. In this mode no electric arcs are generated between electrode and the tissue, as peak voltage is less than 200 V. The end result is shrinkage and desiccation of tissue without charring.

b. Forced coagulation uses electric arcs to achieve deep coagulation. Peak voltages of more than 500V are utilized to obtain this. This is useful in vascular areas.

c. Spray coagulation is a non contact mode which uses intensely modulated high frequency voltages (kV). A wider area of tissue is exposed to current. Its main use is to control bleeding from an inaccessible vessel or to achieve hemostasis in a raw and bleeding area.

For coagulation, current of interrupted wave form of high voltage and low amplitude is used. Cells walls contract using this mode so that there is increased normal clotting. It causes protein denaturation and charring of cells.

2. For cutting, current of continuous wave form of high amplitude and low voltage is used. Heat production causes desiccation of cells due to water evaporation.

3. For blended mode, which can both cut and coagulate, amplitude and voltage are equal.

Modes of Diathermy

1. Monopolar (Fig. 14.1A)
2. Bipolar (Fig. 14.1B)

In monopolar diathermy, current passes from the generator via the active electrode through the patient and returns to electrosurgical unit via a dispersive electrode (patient plate). In order to complete the circuit and to return the current to the electrosurgical unit, a patient plate is always

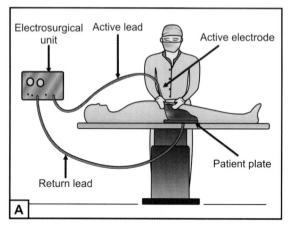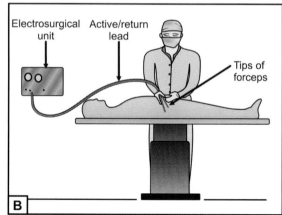

Figs 14.1A and B: Circuit of monopolar diathermy (A) and bipolar diathermy (B)

required. This should be in good contact with the patient's skin over at least 300 square cm or more.

In bipolar mode, current passes from the generator to one prong of bipolar forceps (or scissors), then through the patient tissue caught between the forceps and returns back to generator through the second prong. The current does not therefore pass through the patient's body, as the circuit is completed through the bipolar forceps. This mode does not require a patient plate.

Uses of Bipolar Diathermy

1. When coagulation is required peripherally on an organ with a narrow pedicle, there is risk of channeling the current through the pedicle, leading to thrombosis of vessels, and a deleterious effect on the organ's blood supply. It is therefore safer to use bipolar diathermy in this situation eg circumcision.
2. When pinpoint or microcoagulation is required, e.g. neurosurgery, ophthalmic surgery, or plastic surgery.
3. When patient has a pacemaker *in situ*, in order to avoid problems that may be caused by a unipolar current passing through the heart.

Precautions when using Diathermy

1. Equipment should be checked before use to ensure that it is in good working order. Regular check up and maintenance of electro-surgery units should be performed to prevent injury to the patient and theatre personnel.
2. The diathermy plate or return electrode should be of an appropriate size (300 sq.cm or more). The largest return electrode appropriate to the patient helps to ensure that electrical energy is not concentrated enough to generate significant heat and cause a burn.
3. The diathermy plate should be placed close to the operative site, and on the same side.
4. The diathermy plate should be placed over a vascular and muscular area. Muscle is a better conductor of electricity, and good perfusion promotes electrical conductivity and dissipates heat.
5. If the skin at the site where the plate is to be placed is hairy, it should be shaved, as hair prevents complete plate contact with the patient skin.

6. The diathermy plate should not be placed over a bony prominence, scar tissue, skin over implanted metal prosthesis or areas distal to tourniquets. Bone is not a good conductor of electricity. Tissue perfusion may not be adequate in these areas. The plate can become over heated if placed over an implanted metal prosthesis.

7. The diathermy plate should have a uniform and good body contact to permit the flow of current.

8. There should not be any pooling of blood, body fluids or irrigation fluid near the diathermy plate, as this may lead to loss of contact due to moisture.

9. Patient's jewellery should be removed prior to transfer to theatre as metal jewellery presents a potential risk of burn from directed current.

10. Contact of patient with grounded metal objects, e.g. IV stands, or anesthesia machine should be avoided as they may become an alternate pathway for current leak to ground and can lead to accidental burns.

11. If there is a change in the position of the patient during surgery, the diathermy plate and wire should be re-inspected to make sure that there is no tension on the plate, which can result in reduced plate contact.

12. Alcohol based solutions should be avoided for preoperative skin preparation because they may ignite and increase the risk of a thermo electrical burn.

13. The active diathermy electrode should be placed in an insulated quiver at all times when not in use.

14. The active electrode should have a secure tip. A loose tip may cause a spark. Eschar which built up on the tip prevents the electrode from working safely, and regular cleaning during a surgical procedure may be necessary.

15. Electrosurgical smoke plume presents a potential biological and chemical hazard to both patients and staff. Smoke evacuation systems should be used for all procedures involving use of diathermy.

16. Monopolar units should not be operated in the vicinity of an electrocardiogram electrode (minimum of distance of 15 cm) as they may lead to monitor malfunction.

17. Only the surgeon using the active electrode should active the machine.

18. One should be cautious whilst using diathermy inside bowel. This is because intestinal gas contains the inflammable gases hydrogen and methane which can explode.

Procedure for Starting a Monopolar Diathermy Machine

As the safety of monopolar diathermy depends upon proper placement of the patient plate, and only few diathermy machines have patient plate monitoring systems, one should adhere to the following procedures during startup.

1. Place the patient plate on the patient at appropriate place.
2. Connect the return lead to the patient plate.
3. Switch on diathermy machine, and plate continuity alarm will sound.
4. Connect return electrode to the diathermy machine, so that continuity alarm is silenced.

Hazards of Surgical Diathermy in Minimal Access Surgery (MAS)

Laparoscopic surgery has specific hazards in relation to electrocautery. These hazards are due to the number of instruments and ports within the operative field.

The principal hazards are:
1. *Insulation failure*: This is the commonest cause of burns during MAS, and can be due to

insulation failure, mechanical trauma, and repeated sterilization of instruments or manufacturing flaws. Defects in the tip of the instrument within the view of the laparoscope can cause injury to a non target area, e.g. liver during laparoscopic cholecystectomy. Insulation defects in the shaft of an instrument can cause undetectable injury to any bowel it comes in contact with. Insulation failure at the handle of the instrument can burn the surgeon, or cause electric shock if the surgical glove is defective.

2. *Capacitive Coupling (Fig. 14.2)*: This is a phenomenon where an electrical current in the instrument induces a current in a nearby conductor in spite of intact insulation due to electromagnetic induction. This is because current flowing through an instrument induces an alternating magnetic field around it.

There is increased incidence of capacitive coupling with higher voltages. It is of clinical significance in the following situations:

a. Use of hybrid cannula, i.e. metal cannula within a plastic anchoring cannula.
b. If an insulated electrode is passed through a metal port, there may be induction of current in the port, with up to 70% of current passing through insulated electrode.

c. If an electrode is passed through the working channel of the laparoscope 70% of the current may be induced in the laparoscope.

3. *Direct coupling*: If an activated electrode touches another metal instrument there will be direct transfer of current from activated electrode to metal instrument. Tissues which are in contact with the metal instrument may be injured. Situations where direct coupling can occur are:

a. Touching of an active electrode to the laparoscope.
b. Touching of an active electrode to a metal clip or staple line.

Diathermy and Pacemakers

Diathermy currents can interfere with the working of pacemakers, which may be inhibited during diathermy activation, preventing cardiac pacing during cautery. A pacemaker may revert to a fixed rate of pacing during use of cautery and may require a magnet to reset it. If possible, the use of diathermy in a patient with a pacemaker should be avoided and other sources of energy such as the ultrasonic scalpel should be used.

If it is mandatory to use diathermy in such patients, the following precautions should be taken:

1. Use bipolar mode, avoiding the use of monopolar diathermy.
2. If monopolar cautery is to be used, the patient plate should be sited in such a way that the current path does not pass through the heart or pacemaker.
3. Monitor heart beat throughout the operation.
4. A defibrillator should be available in case of dangerous arrhythmias.
5. Cardiologist should be asked to check pacemaker function prior to surgery.
6. Facilities for inserting a temporary pacemaker should be available.

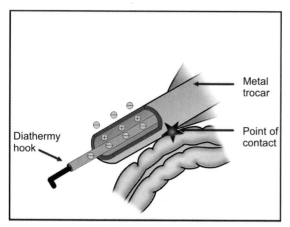

Fig. 14.2: Mechanism of capacitative coupling by diathermy

KEY POINTS

1. Diathermy uses high frequency alternating current (>50 KHz) at which there is no neuromuscular stimulation.
2. Whenever current gets concentrated in a small area heat is generated.
3. One can use diathermy either for cutting or coagulation.
4. Cutting diathermy uses a low voltage, high frequency continuous wave form.
5. Coagulation uses high voltage, low frequency interrupted wave form.
6. Bipolar diathermy is safer than monopolar diathermy because the current does not passes through the patient's body.
7. Faulty position of patient's plate is the most common cause of diathermy burn.
8. Patient's plate must be well in contact with patient body over a well vascularized muscular mass over a minimum area of at least 300 sq. cm.
9. Avoid placing return electrode over scar, bony prominence, or distal to a tourniquet.
10. During laparoscopic surgery additional hazards of diathermy includes direct coupling, insulation failure and capacitive coupling.
11. Do not use monopolar diathermy in a patient with a pace maker.

Dressings and Wound Care

Assessment of Wounds

When assessing wounds it is important to consider:

- Site
- Size
- Shape
- Depth
- Edges
- Surrounding tissues including pulses and sensation.
- Base-slough, eschar, necrotic tissue, granulation tissue
- Malignant change in a chronic ulcer (Marjolin's ulcer).

Microbiology swabs should be sent regularly. The presence of pathological organisms does not necessitate antibiotic treatment unless there is cellulitis or systemic sepsis. Regular dressing changes and debridement prevent bacterial counts from rising.

Necrotic Tissue

Necrotic tissue is devitalized or dead tissue. It is important to debride necrotic tissue to prevent infection, and enhance healing.

Slough

Slough is a mixture of dead cells, fibrin, serous exudate, white blood cells and bacteria. Sloughy wounds correspond to the proliferative stage of

wound healing and it is important to encourage formation of granulation tissue. Large quantities of exudate can macerate surrounding tissues. If large volumes of exudate are present then an absorbent dressing is required. If the wound is dry a dressing that retains moisture should be used.

Granulation Tissue

Granulation tissue is very vascular, resulting in a bright red colour. Dressings should be chosen according to the amount of exudate. Overgranulation prevents epithelialization and healing of the wound. It appears as prominent, friable pink tissue overgrowing a wound edge. It can be treated by application of a silver nitrate pencil.

Epithelialization

Epithelial cells within the basal layer duplicate and migrate across a wound. A low adherence dressing should be used to avoid damaging these tissues. Dressing changes should be kept to a minimum, although it is important not to allow penetration of fluids through a dressing as this increases the risk of infection.

Exudate

Exudate contains leukocytes, enzymes, growth factors and cytokines, all of which are vital in wound healing. There is evidence to suggest that keeping a wound moist with exudate encourages healing.

Principles of Wound Care

When treating any wound it is necessary to consider:
- Nutrition
- Pressure care
- Treat underlying cause
- Drain sepsis/debride wound
- Treat cellulitis
- Clean wound
- Promote healing
- Regular review by same individuals/team
- Documentation of progress.

The Ideal Dressing

The perfect dressing does not exist, however, if it did it would:
- Protect the wound from trauma
- Be impermeable to bacteria
- Allow oxygenation
- Retain moisture
- Be non allergenic
- Would not damage surrounding tissues

Methods of Debridement

Autolytic

Autolytic debridement uses the body's ability to dissolve dead tissue. Dressings are used to enhance water retention in the wound, this traps enzymes, growth factors and other factors involved in healing.

Surgical

Debridement of necrotic tissues can be carried out on the ward during dressing changes. This should not be painful providing there is not extensive inflammation of the surrounding tissues. More extensive debridement may require regional or general anesthetic in theatre.

Biological

Larval therapy involves the application of sterile larvae to the wound, where they selectively digest necrotic tissue. Maggots do not damage healthy tissue.

Enzymatic

A pharmacologically developed version of collagenase has been developed that can aid digestion of necrotic tissue.

Mechanical

Mechanical debridement involves the application of saline soaked gauze to the wound. It is allowed to dry and then removed the next day, removing the superficial layers of tissue.

Types of Dressing

Low Adherence

For example, jelonet, mepitel.
Low adherent dressings allow easy removal without damaging the wound or surrounding tissues.

They allow exudate to seep through to secondary dressing.

They are generally composed of perforated plastics, tulles or textiles, sometimes coated with a low adherent substance such as paraffin wax.

Semi-Permeable

For example, tegaderm, opsite, mepore.
These dressings are permeable to gas and water vapor, however not to fluids or bacteria. These dressings are used in clean, dry or minimally exudating wounds.

Opsite spray is a transparent film dressing spray which is permeable to gas and water vapor, but water-resistant. It is used on areas where a dressing is unlikely to adhere, e.g. flexible areas – fingers, or scalp.

Foam

For example, allevyn, lyofoam.
Foam dressings are composed of hydrophilic polyurethane foam. They are highly absorbent and can absorb heavy volumes of exudate preventing leakage onto surrounding skin.

Hydrocolloid

For example, aquacel, tegasorb, granuflex.
Hydrocolloids contain gel forming agents and form a gel on contact with exudate. They are used for absorbing mild to moderate amounts of exudate and promote autolysis.
They are initially impermeable to exudate and bacteria. However as the gelling process occurs, they are increasingly permeable to exudate.

Hydrogel

For example, intrasite, aquasorb.
Hydrogels are water or glycerin based products, and therefore are gel like in consistency. They are used in cavities to promote autolysis of tissues in necrotic wounds. In dry wounds they are used to provide a moist environment, however, they can macerate surrounding normal tissue. These dressings are not used for exudative wounds as they exhibit poor absorption of exudate. They are nonadherent.

Anti-microbial

For example, Aquacel Ag, inadine, actisorb silver
Anti-microbial dressings contain a topical anti-microbial agent which aims to reduce bacterial load. However, if a wound is overtly infected they will not convert it to a clean wound. Agents used

include silver, iodine and metronidazole. They absorb small amounts of exudate.

Capillary

For example, vacutex.
Capillary dressings consist of a sandwich foam dressing that is highly absorbent and is therefore used for wounds with large amounts of exudate. These dressings damage dry wounds.

Alginate

For example, kaltostat, sorbsan.
Alginates are derived from alginic acid salts in brown seaweed. These dressings are used for heavily exudating wounds as they can absorb five times their weight in water. Alginates should not be used in dry wounds as they will stick, damaging tissue when removed. They are useful for dressing cavities. A secondary covering dressing is required.

Gauze

For example, blue gauze.
Used as a secondary dressing, often on top of low adherence/hydrocolloid dressings to absorb exudates. Also used on top of semi-permeable dressings to provide pressure, reducing the risk of hematoma formation. They should not be applied directly to the wound as they will stick, damaging tissue when removed.

Waterproof

For example, elastoplast.
Waterproof dressings are permeable to gas but not to water vapor, fluids or bacteria. Therefore they maintain a moist wound environment and so can lead to maceration. They are used over surgical wounds where there is a high risk of infection due to wound position (for example over a laparotomy wound next to a stoma).

Vacuum Assisted Closure Device (VAC pump)

The VAC pump applies low negative pressure to draw excess fluid from the wound, promote granulation tissue, aid wound contraction and reduce bacterial counts. A polyurethane ether foam dressing is cut to size and applied to the wound. The suction device is embedded within this and an adhesive, impermeable drape covers the wound and overlaps normal skin. The set up allows equal pressure to be applied across the whole wound. The evacuation tube is connected to an external canister in which the fluid is collected. These devices can be used on an outpatient basis but can also be effective in large wounds in ITU such as laparostomy.

Examples of Dressings

Necrotic Wound e.g. Pressure Sore

The dead tissue in necrotic wounds loses moisture rapidly, and so often becomes hard and dry to touch. In order for healing to occur, this hard, dead, tissue must first be removed, either by surgical debridement, or by rehydrating the tissue thereby promoting autolysis.

Typically a hydrogel, such as intrasite, is applied to the necrotic areas. A barrier cream is used on the edges to prevent maceration of the surrounding tissue. The area is then covered with a semi-permeable dressing and re-inspected every 24 hours.

Sloughy Wound e.g. Ulcer

The presence of a thick layer of slough predisposes to wound infection. Therefore slough should be removed to promote healing, either by mechanical, biological or surgical debridement.

Typically a hydrocolloid dressing is applied to promote autolysis and absorb exudates. For highly exudative wounds an alginate may be used. Gauze is then applied as a secondary dressing.

Granulation Tissue

For granulating wounds a low adherence dressing is used to prevent damage to the delicate tissue. A secondary dressing such as hydrocolloid/alginate is used to absorb exudates. Gauze is then applied to absorb any excess exudate.

Index